Eleanor McKenzie
Consultant Sara Mokone

CHI KUNG

CULTIVATING PERSONAL ENERGY

hamlyn

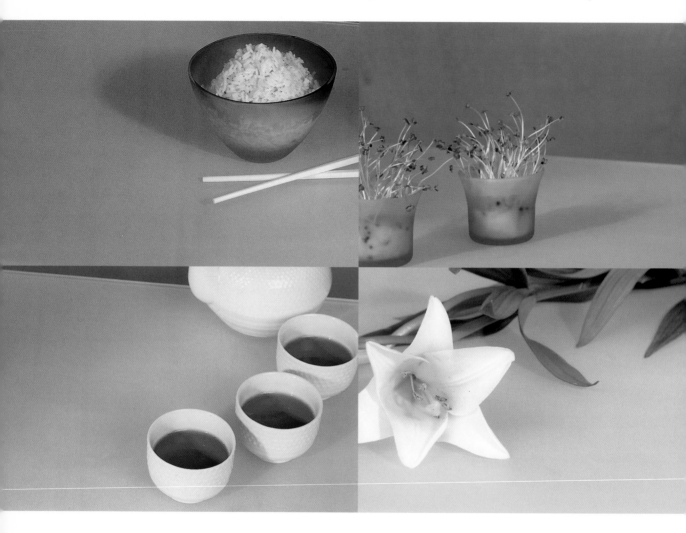

Safety note

It is advisable to check with your doctor before embarking on any exercise programme. Chi kung should not be considered a replacement for professional medical treatment; a physician should be consulted in all matters relating to health and particularly in respect of pregnancy and symptoms which may require diagnosis or medical attention. While the advice and information in this book are believed to be accurate, neither the authors nor the publisher can accept any legal responsibility for any injury sustained while following the suggestions made herein.

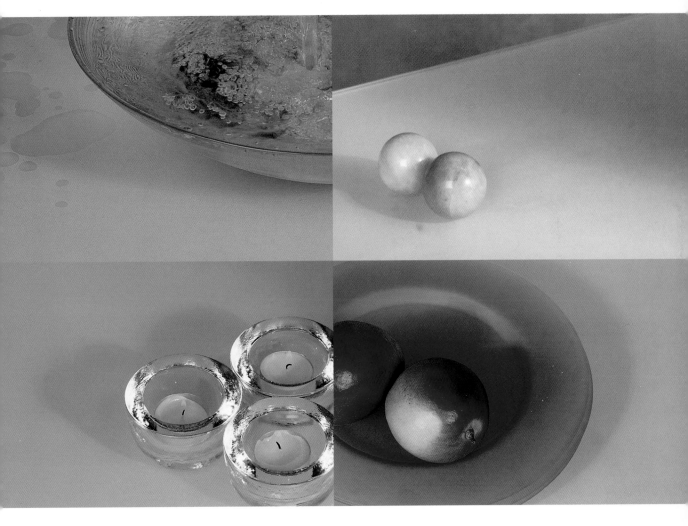

contents

chi kung & the traditions of chinese medicine

The universe is filled with and composed of energy, or *chi*, as is everything within the universe, both animate and inanimate. Mountains, rivers, oceans and stars, as well as animals and humans, are all manifestations of this *chi* in its varying states. Thus, everything in the universe has one source, and because of that everything is connected.

Chi energy is in a constant state of flux: if it wasn't, the sun would not rise and set, the earth would not turn, there would be no seasons and no growth or evolution. Just as the movement of *chi* animates the universe, it animates the processes of the human body. This concept is the foundation of Traditional Chinese Medicine, the tradition to which Chi kung belongs. The aim of its practitioners is to restore and promote the harmonious flow of *chi* in the body, for if the flow of *chi* is impaired, ill health is the result.

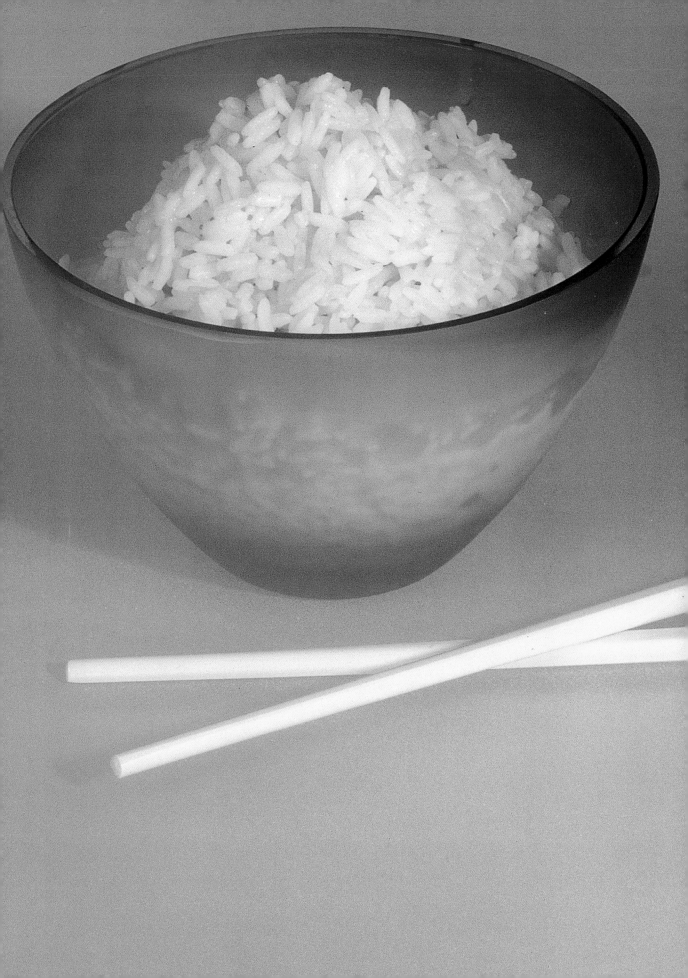

what is chi kung?

Chi kung, or Qigong (pronounced *chee goong*) means 'training the breath' or 'energy cultivation' (*chi* = energy, *gong* = cultivation). At its simplest, the aim of Chi kung is to train the breath in order to promote each person's own healing process.

Chi kung evolved in China, originating even before the advent of written history. Over the centuries, the many spiritual and political movements that developed in China influenced the spread and practice of Chi kung. During the Cultural Revolution it was suppressed, although it continued to flourish in Taiwan. Today, however, its popularity is growing again and it is estimated that over 70 million Chinese practise Chi kung every day. The suppression of Chi kung during the Maoist years in China meant that it remained unknown in the West, where it has only been recognized as a means of solving health problems since the Eighties.

Although there are, reputedly, thousands of forms of Chi kung, it can essentially be divided into two main groups. The first is 'internal' Chi kung, which manipulates the flow of *chi* inside the body. Internal Chi kung has both soft and hard forms, and it can be a martial art like Tai chi and Kung fu, or a soft form that works instead with *chi* internally. It is an art that combines aerobic conditioning, meditation and relaxation, without extreme physical exertion, making it an ideal practice for people of every age and all levels of fitness. It will build up stamina and energy without the risk of physical damage sometimes associated with working out at a gym, and as it does not require any equipment, you can practise it any time, anywhere. The transfer of *chi* is similar to techniques such as therapeutic touch or spiritual healing.

So broad is the definition of Chi kung that spontaneous dancing, walking and other physical activities are all forms of it, but to practise a series of specific Chi kung exercises means consciously choosing to cultivate your personal energy. This book is primarily concerned with the conscious use of Chi kung to control the flow of *chi* into and out of, as well as within, the body.

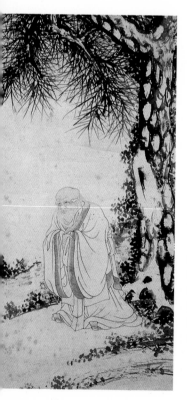

left   The legendary Lao Tzu, founder of Taoism, in a 16th-century Chinese painting by Quan Gi. The Taoist philosophy forms the basis of Chi kung.

right   An 18th-century detail from an illustration of the death of Buddha, National Museum, Bankok. There are thousands of varieties of Chi kung, many of which are closely related to Buddhism.

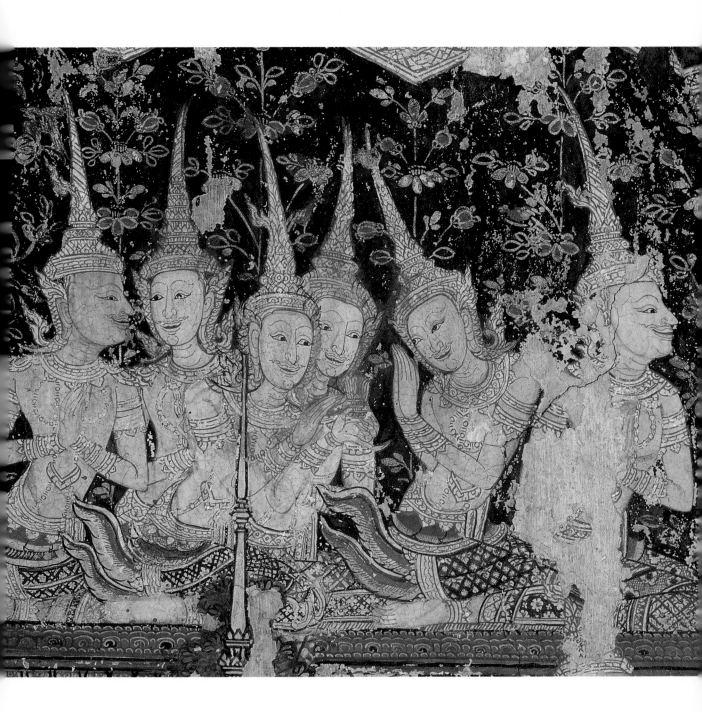

a short history of traditional chinese medicine

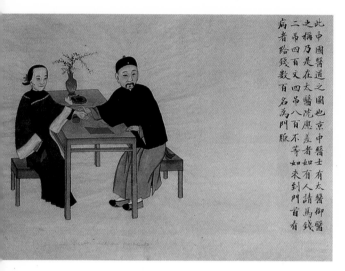

above A 19th-century water-colour by Zhou Pei Qun showing a Chinese physician taking a woman's pulse. Pulse-taking is a fundamental part of diagnosis in Traditional Chinese Medicine.

Chi kung is one of the pillars of Traditional Chinese Medicine (TCM). In order to appreciate the way in which it can be used to prevent ill health and to relieve the symptoms of existing illnesses, it is useful to have a basic knowledge of the principles that unite all the forms of TCM. These are most famously enshrined in what is known as the *Yellow Emperor's Classic of Internal Medicine*, or the *Nei Jing*. One of the best-known Chinese medical texts, it is thought to have been written in the third century BC. Amazingly, not only is it still in print, it is still used by practitioners of Chinese medicine. This gives you some idea of the antiquity of the Chinese system of medicine. It also indicates that current practitioners have found that the theories of health promotion and principles of diagnostic practice established in the period 722–221 BC are still relevant today.

The fundamental principles of health preservation, which are systematically discussed in the *Yellow Emperor's Classic*, are based on ancient observations of the natural world and the laws governing it. Our ancestors saw that everything on earth progresses through a cycle of birth, growth, decline and finally death. This is most obvious in plants, animals and humans, but even mountains and deserts are constantly changing. For example, Mount Everest, is not the same mountain that it was a thousand years ago – it is not even the same mountain that it was yesterday, for it is constantly going through a cycle of degeneration and regeneration caused by the elemental forces of sun, wind, rain and snow.

Even the human body renews itself on a daily basis. Scientists have discovered that cell renewal occurs in every part of the body but at different rates. So, as in the rest of nature, the body you have today is slightly different from the one you had yesterday. It is this process that allows us to stay healthy and to rid the body of toxins and environmental pollutants that damage our cells. It is when this process of renewal is disturbed in some way that illness occurs. From the perspective of TCM, the process is disturbed because the flow of *chi* has been interrupted, and the practitioner's first aim is to restore balance and harmony to the flow of *chi* so that cellular renewal returns to its ideal rate.

This cycle of birth and death is a universal, unchangeable law and means we cannot live forever, despite the progression of science. Yet our ancestors in various cultures saw that if we could understand the laws governing this cycle we could use them to enjoy healthier and longer lives. The average human lifespan in the developed world is now longer than ever, due to improved living conditions, better nutrition, cleaner water and medical advances. However, according to the principles of Chinese medicine, we could extend our lifespans even more, simply by looking after our own energy or *chi*. This is one of the key principles of all forms of TCM.

chi energy

Chi is a concept that appears in many cultures under a different name including *prana* in Hindu tradition and the 'quantum field' in modern physics. *Chi* is also understood as the principle of change, the eternal flux of the universe. It is a difficult term to explain and the Chinese dictionary definition shows it has changed through time. Originally the symbol for 'fire' was used, equating energy with warmth; then it was changed to the symbol for 'no fire', representing the balance of opposites. The present symbol is a grain of rice with air or steam rising above it. We can interpret this symbolically: the body requires food and air (rice and steam) and breathing brings the warm steam to 'cook' the rice, so that we digest the food.

The universe is composed of constantly moving and changing *chi* energy. This is the fundamental concept upon which all the other principles of TCM hang. However, *chi* is not uniform. In matter it manifests in different degrees of density – a brick is denser than the human hand, for example, yet masters of Chi kung and of martial arts like Kung fu can smash a brick with their hand. They can do this because they have spent years refining their intuitive understanding of *chi* at the physical, mental and spiritual levels.

Also, not all *chi* is nourishing energy, but this does not mean that it should be seen in a negative light – negative *chi* is not the same as bad *chi*. Positive, negative and neutral *chi* are descriptions more akin to the way in which physics describes the objective properties of electricity.

For good health, *chi* must flow harmoniously and also be balanced. Similarly, in the home, a Feng shui practitioner will also investigate the flow of *chi* into and through the house. As with the body, anything that negatively affects the flow of *chi* has to be removed or, if *chi* is stagnant, action is taken to restore its circulation.

Therefore the universal principles of *chi*, as understood by the Chinese for thousands of years, can be applied in an infinite number of ways. From preserving health, to increasing good fortune or divining the future, they all rest on the understanding that the universe is *chi* energy.

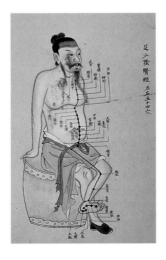

below An ancient acupuncture chart. The use of acupuncure is now widespread in the West and is often recommended by orthodox physicians to ease a variety of conditions.

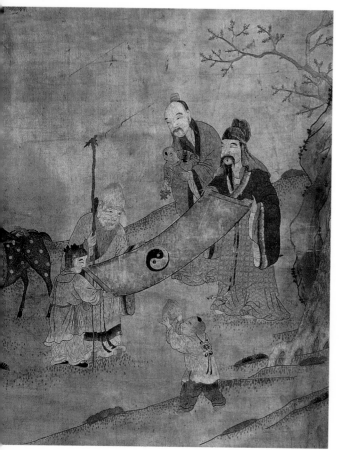

above Young and old study the
yin yang symbol in this 17th-
century Chinese painting. This
ancient concept involves the
perfect balance of two opposites
– usually identified as male
and female.

yin and yang

Another fundamental principle of Chinese philosophy and
medicine is the concept of yin and yang. Although yin and
yang are often thought of as opposites, there is always an
element of yin in yang and vice versa. That is why, in the
well-known Chinese yin/yang symbol, there is a dot of white
yang within the black yin and a black dot of yin within the
white yang.

Yin is primarily associated with the feminine and the yang
with masculine. In Chinese philosophy everything in the
universe can be classified as being either yin or yang, but
neither can exist without the other. For example, there would
be no night (yin) without day (yang) and no male (yang)
without female (yin). The following list gives a few examples
of the attributes of each, but it is by no means exhaustive.

Yin	Yang
Female	Male
Dark/night	Light/day
Cold	Heat
Soft	Hard
Winter	Summer
Inner	Outer
Earth	Sky
Moon	Sun
Negative	Positive
Passive	Active

TCM also classifies areas of the body, body processes and
the symptoms of ill health as being either yin or yang, and
illness itself is considered to be the result of a yin/yang
imbalance. Some of the specific areas of the body and
physical symptoms that are seen as either yin or yang are
given below:

Yin area	Yang area
Interior	Surface
Front	Back
Blood	*Chi* energy

Yin symptom	Yang symptom
Retiring	Advancing
Cold skin	Hot skin
Low temperature	High temperature
Shivering	Feverish
Chronic	Acute
Moist	Dry

Thus, symptoms classified as yang have qualities associated with other yang attributes. For example, heat or high temperature and dryness are symptoms associated with yang imbalance in the body and they also correspond to yang qualities in the world around us, if you compare the two lists.

The yin/yang symbol is the basis of the Chinese compass, the *Pa kua*, with its eight trigrams as used in Feng shui. The eight trigrams can then be expanded to form the 64 hexagrams of the *I Ching*, the *Book of Changes*, used for the purpose of divination. In short, for the Chinese, the yin/yang symbol represents all their spiritual and philosophical beliefs in one image.

the five elements

Wood – spring, liver and gall bladder

Fire – summer, heart and small intestine

Earth – late summer, spleen and stomach

Metal – autumn, lungs and large intestine

Water – winter, kidneys and bladder

As well as the concepts of *chi* and yin and yang, the Five Elements, sometimes referred to as 'phases of change' are also fundamental to TCM. These elements are, fire, water, wood, metal and earth, and they correspond to the organs of the body and the seasons (see left).

An individual's personality will also display the characteristics of one of the five elements; a Chinese medical practitioner will calculate your dominant element and use this information in assessing the correct treatment for you.

Personality types

Wood – purposeful, active, sometimes domineering, should avoid windy places

Fire – intuitive and communicative, seeks excitement and is easily bored, should avoid heat

Earth – loyal and fond of company, good attention to detail but can be stubborn, should avoid damp

Metal – organized, controlling, discriminating and appreciates quality, should avoid dryness

Water – imaginative, clever, secretive, needs protection, should avoid cold

The Five Elements also relate to sounds, tastes and compass directions, and most books devoted to Chinese medicine or philosophy show these correspondences in full. Each of the elements helps or hinders the others, something that a TCM practitioner fully understands. The Five Elements concept plays a major part in every application of Chinese philosophy and together with yin and yang provides a comprehensive and holistic view of the universe and everything in it.

the meridians

The meridians are the invisible channels that conduct *chi* around the body, and are a primary feature of the Chinese anatomy of energy. Although they are considered to be separate from all the other anatomical systems, for example the nervous or lymphatic systems, they run in parallel to these systems and are complementary to them. Thus, if the *chi* that flows along the meridians is blocked or weakened, or if the flow is reversed, this will eventually manifest as physical and emotional imbalance.

Such a concept can be explained in simple terms of energy and matter. Energy vibrates at a higher frequency than matter and most human eyesight is unable to see it. Western science, as well as the ancient Chinese and Hindu scientific systems, suggests that energy, vibrating at a higher rate, has an effect on matter, vibrating at a much lower rate. Translated into TCM terms, matter – or the body – is affected by energy or *chi*. Illness is therefore the result of a primary imbalance in the body's energy system, which in Chinese medicine depends on the flow of *chi* through the meridians (or, in Hindu tradition, through the *chakras*, or energy centres of the body).

There are a total of 35 meridians in the system, conduct-ing *chi* through the body. Within these there are 12 major meridians, 8 extra meridians and 15 collateral channels. It is along the major meridians and the Governor and Conception channels, which are extra meridians, that the 'acupoints' are found. These are the points used in acupuncture and acu-pressure to effect changes in the energy system.

The 12 major meridians are each related to a specific organ in the body, although not to the 'physical' organ itself, but rather to its function. In the West, each one is named after its relevant organs – heart, lungs, kidneys, and so on. Each is also related to many other aspects of the person, both physical and emotional. Other correspondences link the main meridians with particular elements. The stomach and spleen meridians, for example, are linked with the element of Earth, and they are also connected with the colour yellow, with sympathy (emotion), sweetness (taste), flesh (tissue) and dampness (climate).

Apart from the 12 major meridians, the Governor and Conception channels are the only meridians that have acupoints on them. The Governor channel, which has 28 points, runs up the centre of the back and over the top of the head, ending on the upper lip. The Conception channel, with 24 points, runs up the centre front, ending at the bottom lip. As part of the Eight Extra Meridians or vessels, these chan-nels are considered to be reservoirs of energy which can be drawn on whenever there is a deficiency. Some of the very central exercises of Chi kung involve circulating *chi* through the Governor and Conception channels, also known as the Microcosmic Orbit.

If an imbalance arises in the body's energy system, the aim of TCM is to correct this by restoring the proper flow of *chi* through the meridians. For this the acupuncturist uses needles at relevant points on the meridians. In Feng shui, a plant or ornament is placed to have the same effect. In Chi kung, the exercises perform these different functions. Some increase the quantity of *chi* coming into the body through the use of breath, while others improve the circulation of the *chi* already in the body or aim to improve the *chi* in particular organs, all of which have their own type of energy.

Of course, if we all knew how to look after our energy in a way that prevented physical symptoms from manifesting, we would never be ill – and in TCM, that is precisely the function of Chi kung.

applying the principles

Traditional Chinese Medicine covers a wide number of treat-ment methods, the main ones being:

- Acupuncture and moxibustion
- Acupressure
- Herbal medicine
- Tui na massage
- Chi kung or Qigong
- Tai chi or Taijiquan
- Feng shui

In the West, the conventional medical view puts forward the belief that, while the symptoms of a disease may vary in severity between individuals, the physiological cause is always the same. From this point of view, it is logical, there-fore, that the same treatment approach is taken with each person, only adjusting it slightly according to the mildness or severity of the symptoms. However, this does not allow for the physical, emotional and spiritual uniqueness of the individual who is being treated.

For example, a person with arthritis who is being treated by conventional medicine will be given the same drug treat-ment as other arthritis sufferers. TCM practitioners, on the other hand, will consider the whole person in making a diagnosis, not just their physical symptoms. They will take various pulses, inspect the tongue to find out how the whole body is working and which organs are deficient in energy and look at the general appearance and the colour of the skin. They will also listen to the person's voice and how they speak, enquire about sleeping patterns, eating and drinking patterns, preferences for hot or cold and other lifestyle and emotional questions. It is from all these simple observations that they will find the cause of the person's physical symptoms.

Oriental medicine is no longer unfamiliar to Westerners, many of whom will have experienced one of the forms of treatment themselves. Many Chinese herbalists have premises on local high streets, and acupuncture is widely used or recommended by orthodox medical practitioners, particularly for pain relief. Although these therapies are different, they are all based on the same fundamental principles, and on a view that sees every person as unique and requiring a unique diagnosis and form of treatment. Tai chi and Chi kung classes are also widely available and are popular across all age groups.

how chi kung works

Using gentle stretching exercises combined with breathing techniques and visualization, Chi kung balances the flow of *chi* energy through the meridians, thereby promoting the health of the physical organs as well as mind and spirit. As a strand of TCM, the primary aim of Chi kung is to prevent disease and promote longevity. That is why the Chinese consider it to be a 'national treasure'. In contrast, Western medicine has developed as a means of curing disease, and does not include a systematic method for preventing it. As a result, we expect doctors to perform miracles and hand ourselves over to them. To practise Chi kung regularly is to empower ourselves by taking control of our own life force, so we can perform our own miracles.

There are thousands of varieties of Chi kung, stemming from five main traditions: Taoist, Buddhist, Confucian, martial arts and medical, but of these, the Taoist philosophy forms the roots of Chi kung. This is a philosophy based on an organic view of the world. The early Taoists were also scientists, as they constructed both scientific and philosophical theories from their observation of the natural world. They observed the connections between the movement of the planets, the seasons, and the cycles of all plant and animal life. The most famous exposition of Taoist thought is the *Tao Te Ching*, a text which is attributed to Lao Tzu, the most famous Taoist sage. In a passage from the *Tao Te Ching* (see right), the Tao is described thus:

The Tao is the origin of the One,

The One created the two,

The two formed the three.

From the three came forth all life.

(Lao Tzu, *Tao Te Ching*)

The 'two' referred to in the previous passage from the *Tao Te Ching* are yin and yang, and the 'three' are heaven, earth and man. Only the Tao is undefined: it has no qualities, it is simply a way of living.

Taoism is an exquisitely refined philosophical system that has many aspects, but its core idea, as exemplified above, is that the Tao is the origin of everything and that our aim in life is to be in harmony with the Tao. But the Tao is something that is transcendent. The Tao simply *is*, and cannot be defined. Therefore, being in harmony with the Tao is a state of consciousness. However, it is a state of consciousness beyond the everyday, and when you are one with the Tao you will not know it, you will simply *be* it. This concept is not so very different from that found in other philosophies which claim the pursuit of enlightenment as the chief aim of every individual's life. In Hinduism, yoga – which includes many more practices than the *asanas* of Hatha yoga, the most well-known form in the West – is the path to transcendence. For Taoists, practising Chi kung is a way of achieving that state of consciousness.

For Chi kung is more than a set of physical exercises, in the same way that Hatha yoga, in its entirety, is more than just the discipline of yoga. Chi kung is also a way of meditation; which, like meditation forms in other systems, such as Vipassana, a Theravada Buddhist meditation technique which utilizes the breath to achieve insight, uses breath and visualization to alter and expand consciousness. When we expand our consciousness, using even something as apparently simple as our breath, we alter first our perception of our own lives, then alter of our perceptions of the lives of others. The more frequently we do this, the more our lives change and progress without our ever having consciously to will or control the changes. Every aspect of our life is touched by this, including our bodies. As we start to move with the flow of life, our bodies and minds become soft and supple, bending and unresisting. We then experience our true power through the harmony of physical health and emotional joy.

While there are different forms of Chi kung, all forms have common characteristics. From this point of view, it might be said that the differences between forms are merely stylistic, but as they all have a common purpose the ultimate effect is the same. This may be compared to music. Most musical styles are created from a basic eight-note scale, yet that scale is the source of opera, jazz and rock In the same way, all forms of Chi kung are simply variations on a theme.

The characteristics shared by all forms of Chi kung are:

- Awareness of heaven, earth and man and the movement of energy in the body
- Control of posture, breathing and visualization
- Relaxation
- Static Chi kung involves 'internal' practices, such as breathing and standing exercises, and is a form of meditation
- Dynamic Chi kung, involving practices that require external movement of the body
- Use of the meridian system and acupoints
- Use of the Triple Heaters or Three *Dantian*, the three main energy centres in the upper, middle and lower body
- Strengthening of the body systems, such as the endocrine and the nervous systems, as well as the organs and tissues.

practising chi kung

Chi kung cultivates energy through regular practice and experience of the energy – as an analogy, you can describe a strawberry in words, but it is only by eating one that you can experience what the word 'strawberry' actually means. In contrast to the fast pace of Western life and the 'instant-fix' Western attitude, Chi kung relies on dedication and steady commitment. To fully appreciate the many benefits of Chi kung, practitioners have to step outside the 'fast is good' attitude and adopt instead a slow but sure approach to seeing results.

Chi kung can bring about rejuvenation and longevity, both of which are highly desirable, but not after practising for just one week. The effects of Chi kung build up over time. What is required is patience and a relaxed attitude. Practising Chi kung weekly, or daily as you build up your practice, will bring incredible benefits, but you will only appreciate the benefits if you make your practice regular – even if that is only once a week.

Chi kung is an excellent method of treating many chronic illnesses such as hypertension and multiple sclerosis, and is now widely used for this purpose in Chinese hospitals. It is also commonly used for lowering blood pressure, improving circulation, building the immune system and treating asthma and migraines. However, the practice of Chi kung is primarily used for the prevention of ill health. This book shows you how a few easily learnt exercises, practised regularly, can improve the quality of your life and keep you free of sickness and feeling young.

The exercises in this book are taught to medical students in China and are based on principles researched in China over the last 20 years. Many Chi kung classes teach a particular form of Chi kung but, when properly followed, all forms lead not just to excellent physical and mental health, but ultimately to spiritual enlightenment as well. Some teachers may expect their students to stick to a particular form, and to follow the philosophy of that school. As this book is a general introduction to Chi kung, it focuses on exercises that primarily have the capacity to improve basic physical health and general mental relaxation. Those who want to progress to using the more advanced Chi kung techniques that allow practitioners to transmit *chi* externally, and extend their psychic abilities, should find a reputable teacher.

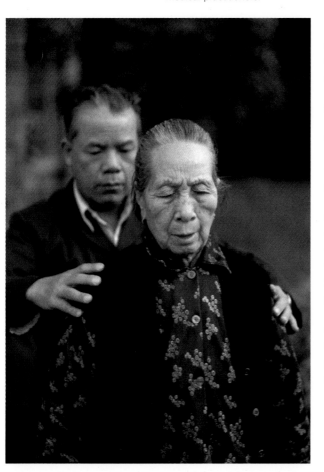

below Healing with Chi kung, Guangzhou, China. Chi kung is revered for its healing properties in China and is commonly used for treating numerous ailments by orthodox medical practitioners.

choosing a chi kung class

All books and videos on Chi kung, are essentially supplements to practical experience – they are not a substitute for attending Chi kung classes. When you attend classes you are likely to want to explore the subject beyond the class, try out different postures or explore other teachers' theories, and you will use books or videos to do that. But your practice is less likely to be successful if you learn alone and rely solely on books and videos. This is true of the learning experience in general and particularly true of any subject that requires physical participation, where experience will teach you more than theory.

By attending a class you will benefit from the experience of the teacher, who can address your own particular problems and queries. If you need healing, choose a teacher who has a background in TCM. This is important. For example, if you have high or low blood pressure, or joint or spinal problems, the teacher will advise you on the best way to approach your specific problem, the best exercises for you to use, and the way to do them that will be comfortable for you. This will make you feel more confident about your practice and you will have comfort in knowing that the teacher is there to give you personal help, although this may be somewhat limited by the time available within the class. However, a good teacher, of any subject, knows how to make time and recognizes when people in the class require individual attention.

Chi kung classes are usually advertised in specialist health or New Age magazines and in local newspapers. You will probably not be able to tell from the advertisement what type of approach the teacher takes. Some Chi kung practitioners teach only a set form, while others combine forms, as shown in this book, and provide a broader approach. The general approach is probably more useful for complete beginners, since it will allow you to understand the basics before you move on.

If you want to know what the teacher's approach is, ask them before you start the class. For example, if you are a beginner, establish that it is a class suitable for beginners. Use your intuition about the information the teacher gives you and ask them about their training and how long they have been practising and teaching. You should also be aware that teachers taught by Chinese masters and following a Chinese style of teaching may have a different style to that in the West. To Westerners, it will appear more rigid and formal, and it is likely that there will be little, if any, focus on individual needs in the class. This is a purely cultural difference and while some Westerners are happy with it, others are not.

Also, as in many other spheres of learning, there are Chi kung masters or teachers who expect their students to revere them. They may also deliberately withhold knowledge from their students in order to maintain their position of superiority. They have their reasons for adopting this attitude, but it is not in the spirit of Chi kung, nor can it be attributed to cultural differences. Of course, there is only so much you can find out from a conversation, but if what you hear sounds good, then try a few sessions of the class. Once you begin a class you will know if it is the right class for you. Again, follow your feelings. Do you feel you can trust the teacher? Are you comfortable with them and do you feel respect for them? Are they themselves a good advertisement for Chi kung?

Another very good reason for joining a class is that there are even more benefits to be had from practising Chi kung in a group. On one level, it is simply good for us to be in company, to meet new people and, ideally, to share experiences. That is health-enhancing in itself. On another level, when several people practise Chi kung together, they all benefit from each other's *chi* energy. People in the class feeling low in energy or unwell can benefit from the energy of those who are stronger at that moment. This does not mean that the stronger people are losing *chi* to the weaker people; it is rather that the quality and quantity of energy in the class becomes balanced, and everyone, no matter what their *chi* level is, makes a contribution to the shared pool of energy. Although it is better not to do Chi kung exercises when you are either ill or emotionally upset, if you are just feeling a bit tired or down, taking part in a class will always lift your energy and spirits.

Finally, Chi kung is still in its infancy in the West and classes are not yet widely available. If you cannot find a Chi kung class that is convenient for you, you might consider taking a Tai chi class instead. Tai chi is more established and the basic exercises have the same roots as those in Chi kung. If you are not interested in the martial arts aspect of Tai chi, you can leave that out of your personal practice and still have the health benefits of harmonizing your *chi*.

right Dawn exercise regime, Beijing. In China, Chi kung classes often involve large numbers of people in an open-air setting.

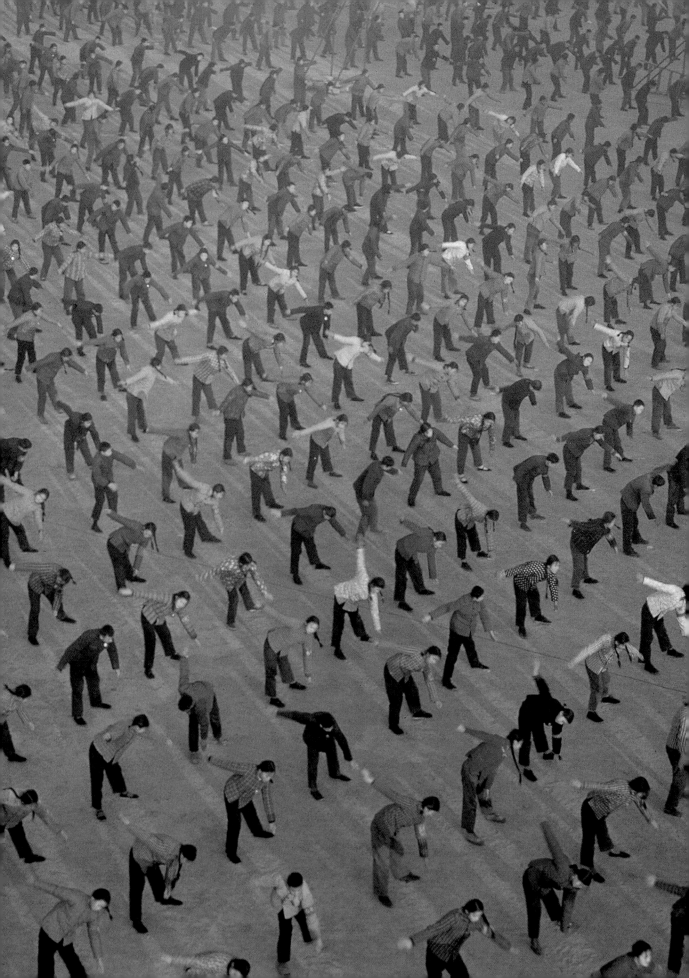

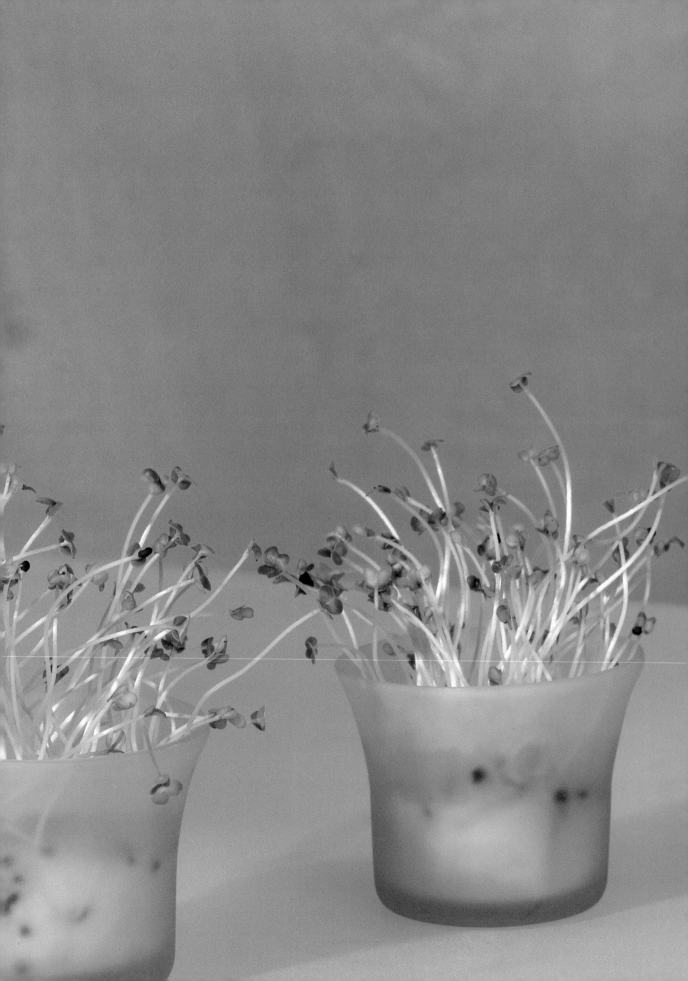

systems of the human body

Anatomy describes the structure of a system and physiology describes how that system works. In TCM and Chi kung, *chi* in the human body has its own anatomy and physiology, which is often referred to as 'energy anatomy' and 'energy physiology'. The mechanism that controls the flow of energy in the energy anatomy is the meridian system, while the principles of yin and yang, the process of change and natural cycles are the laws on which the energy physiology is based.

While Western medicine considers physiological processes in great detail, Chinese medicine regards the patient as a unity of body, mind and spirit and sees the body as a miniature cosmos. However, since the human body is universally the same, it seems logical that both approaches are describing similar things, albeit in very different ways.

the musculo-skeletal structure

The musculo-skeletal system consists of the muscles, bones, ligaments and joints of the body. The bones of the skeleton are the foundation of the system, but not all the bones are constructed in the same way. Some bones, particularly long ones such as the femur or thigh bone, have a central cavity that is filled with bone marrow. This contains tissue that produces our red and white blood cells. The rest of the bones in the skeleton have an inner construction similar to a honeycomb with a hard outer layer. The whole skeleton is connected by a series of joints, the major ones being the ball and socket joints of the hips and shoulders, which allow more flexible movement than the knee or elbow joints, for example. Apart from providing the framework on which the rest of the body is constructed, the main task of the skeletal system is to allow body movement.

One of the main functions of the muscles is to protect the skeleton. Muscles are composed of muscle fibre and there are two types: involuntary and voluntary. The heart, which is both a muscle and a major organ, is an involuntary muscle, as is the digestive tract. This means that we do not consciously control them. The voluntary muscles, such as those in the arms and legs, for example, are primarily used to control all our external movements, such as walking. These muscles are under our control, and we are constantly sending them instructions about the movements we want to make, causing them to contract and relax. The joints of the skeleton that are also involved in these external movements are protected by the ligaments, which consists of a type of flexible tissue.

Medical conditions or injury associated with the musculo-skeletal system are ones that primarily inhibit movement. One common problem is damage to the joints and ligaments through injury or simple wear and tear. But perhaps the most common problem of all is backache, followed by all forms of arthritis. Backache results from a number of physical causes, such as muscle and ligament damage, a slipped disc or trapped nerves, but it can also be caused by emotional trauma. Another problem, which particularly affects women and elderly people, is osteoporosis, or thinning bones.

These problems can be prevented through the practice of Chi kung, and it can also help to restore muscle and bone function through specific exercises that do not require excessive movement.

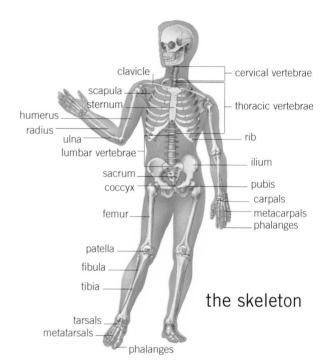

clavicle
cervical vertebrae
scapula
sternum
thoracic vertebrae
humerus
radius
ulna
rib
lumbar vertebrae
ilium
sacrum
coccyx
pubis
carpals
metacarpals
femur
phalanges
patella
fibula
tibia

the skeleton

tarsals
metatarsals
phalanges

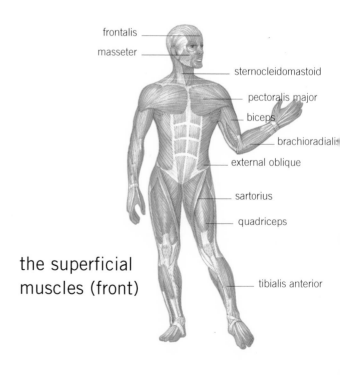

frontalis
masseter
sternocleidomastoid
pectoralis major
biceps
brachioradialis
external oblique
sartorius
quadriceps

the superficial muscles (front)

tibialis anterior

the endocrine system

The function of the endocrine system is to secrete the chemicals known as hormones throughout the body via the bloodstream and in so to regulate the action of both organs and tissues. Hormones also help the body to fight infection, to react to stress and are essential for the reproduction process. Problems with the endocrine system lead to diseases that are strongly suggestive of the concept of imbalance – diabetes, hypothyroidism and hyperthyroidism and infertility, all of which are caused by hormone levels being either too high or too low.

1 Ovaries (connected to the root *chakra*)

2 Pancreas (connected to the solar plexus *chakra*)

3 Adrenal glands (connected to the sacral *chakra*)

4 Thymus gland (connected to the heart *chakra*)

5 Thyroid and parathyroid glands (connected to the throat *chakra*)

6 Pituitary gland (connected to the brow *chakra*)

7 Pineal gland (connected to the crown *chakra*)

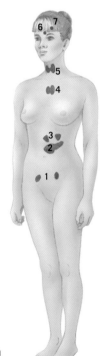

the endocrine system

The endocrine system is made up of the following glands:

• the pituitary
• the pineal
• the thyroid and parathyroids ,
• the thymus
• the islets of Langerhans in the pancreas
• the adrenals
• the gonads in men and the ovaries in women.

The pituitary gland – the main gland of the endocrine system which resides in the brain along with the pineal gland, is thought to secrete melatonin and control our internal body clock. The pituitary coordinates all the other glands in the system and also produces the hormones that influence growth, urine production and uterine contractions. The thyroid gland, which is in the neck, controls metabolism. When it is not secreting enough of the hormone thyroxine, hypothyroidism occurs. This is characterized by sluggishness, weight gain, coldness and depression. When too much thyroxine is secreted, hyperthyroidism occurs, characterized by symptoms such as weight loss, sweating and palpitations of the heart. The parathyroids, located on each lobe of the main gland, are essential for the maintenance of healthy bones, nerves and muscles, and act to balance levels of calcium and phosphorus in the body.

The thymus, located in the chest cavity near the heart, is essential for the maintenance of a healthy immune system. The islets of Langerhans are in the pancreas and are responsible for the secretion of insulin and glucogen to maintain correct levels of glucose in the blood, an imbalance of which results in diabetes mellitus. The adrenal glands lie above the kidneys. They produce two main types of hormone: the outer layer produces steroid hormones that control salt, sugar and water concentration in the body, while the inner layer produces the adrenalin necessary to stimulate the 'fight or flight' reaction. The gonads and ovaries secrete hormones necessary for reproduction. Women suffering from an imbalance here will manifest symptoms varying from infertility to irregular menstruation and PMS.

Chi kung exercises can help to maintain the delicate balance of this system and they can also rectify specific problems that arise, such as diabetes.

the nervous system
& the major organs

While the endocrine system orchestrates the activities of organs and tissues via chemical messengers, the nervous system is the body's control and communications centre. The central nervous system is situated in the brain and spinal cord and controls our conscious and unconscious functions, while the peripheral nervous system consists of both sensory and motor nerves that send messages to the central system.

The brain itself consists of a right and left hemisphere. The right hemisphere controls the motor functions of the left side of the body and vice versa. The right hemisphere also controls feelings and imagination, while the left controls speech and logic, hence creative people are often said to be very 'right-brained'. Our automatic functions, such as breathing, are controlled by the brain stem and our coordination is controlled by the cerebellum.

The common problems involving the nervous system are those that are associated with the brain area; stroke or cerebral haemorrhage, as a result of an arterial blood clot in the cerebrum, when not fatal, causes paralysis, usually on the side of the body controlled by the brain hemisphere where the haemorrhage occurs. Migraine is another problem, as is meningitis. Psychological problems such as depression, anxiety and insomnia are also associated with the nervous system and are sometimes caused by chemical imbalance in the brain.

the autonomic nervous system

The musculo-skeletal, endocrine and nervous systems, the respiratory, circulatory and digestive systems, are interconnected so that the body works harmoniously. The system which demonstrates that connection and interdependence, and which is of particular interest to Chi kung practitioners, is the autonomic nervous system, which includes parts of the peripheral and central nervous systems and controls functions which occur without conscious effort.

The autonomic nervous system is composed of two parts that act together – the sympathetic and parasympathetic. These are responsible for regulating heartbeat, blood pressure, breathing rate and body temperature, amongst other activities. Parts of the system also respond to emotional stress and prepare the body for strenuous physical activity.

The sympathetic system deals with involuntary body functions such as heartbeat and breathing. It is also responsible for activating the adrenal glands in response to stress, and prepares the body for the 'fight or flight' syndrome. Conversely, the parasympathetic system is most active when the body is in a relaxed state, and it also helps to return the body to a relaxed state following a stressful episode. In this way the two systems act to provide balance. For example, some organs contain nerve fibres from both systems. The sympathetic nerves carry impulses that activate the organ while the parasympathetic impulses inhibit it. So during an emergency, for instance, the sympathetic system will increase the activity of the heart and lungs, and when the emergency is over, the parasympathetic will slow them down again.

These two systems need to be balanced to maintain good health. If the sympathetic system is constantly overused as modern living imposes more stress upon us, it works against that balance. That is why a technique like Chi kung is invaluable in utilizing the parasympathetic system so our bodies can rest and repair themselves.

Another technique that helps to control the autonomic nervous system is autogenic training. This is a form of deep relaxation that teaches you to control the two systems and consciously switch between them; it has been shown to bring the two hemispheres of the brain into a balanced state that is conducive to self-healing.

the human anatomy

1 Cerebral cortex connected to the seventh *chakra*

2 Medulla oblongata connected to the sixth *chakra*

3 Upper lungs connected to the fifth *chakra*

4 Heart connected to the fourth *chakra*

5 Lower lungs connected to the fourth *chakra*

6 Liver connected to the third *chakra*

7 Spleen connected to the third *chakra*

8 Stomach connected to the third *chakra*

9 Kidneys connected to the second *chakra*

10 Pancreas connected to the third *chakra*

11 Small intestine connected to the second *chakra*

12 Large intestines connected to the second *chakra*

13 Bladder connected to the second *chakra*

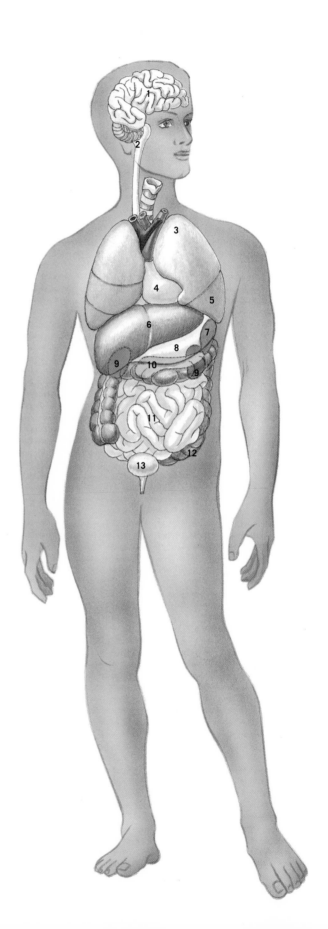

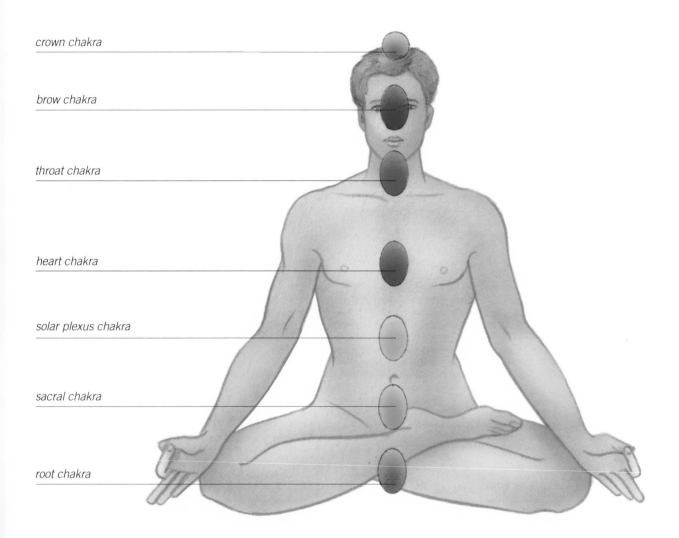

crown chakra

brow chakra

throat chakra

heart chakra

solar plexus chakra

sacral chakra

root chakra

the chakras

comparing eastern & western body systems

Chi kung is a method of cultivating and consciously controlling the higher form of energy or vital essence known as *chi*, regulating its balance and flow in the energy anatomy. While we can learn and understand the Chinese concept of *chi*, we primarily think in terms of our own biomedical system, and we rightly have a cultural need to understand other systems in relationship to our own. Sometimes a relationship can be formed and sometimes not, since the medical approaches originating in the East, including India, are based on spiritual doctrines. In contrast, Western medicine, with its philosophical roots in the scientific materialism of the 17th century, most emphatically has no spiritual dimension for historical reasons. Therefore, while it is possible to make some comparisons in biomedical terms, you have to remember that the Oriental medical systems also see the body as a major path to union with God or the divine, while the Western biomedical system actually grew out of denying God's influence on matter.

The *chakra* system of Hindu philosophy provides an example of the way in which Eastern and Western systems can be compared although such comparisons are not exact. There are seven *chakras*, or energy centres, in the *chakra* system, which influence the health of the physical body through the invisible etheric or energy body in which the *chakras* are located. This etheric body vibrates at a higher frequency than the dense, lower-frequency physical body. Imbalances in the higher frequency flow down to the physical, creating disease there. Imbalance in a *chakra* can manifest as a slowing of the speed at which it spins, corresponding to under-functioning in the physical organs, or a *chakra* may spin too fast and open too wide, also leading to physical and emotional problems.

This concept of the energy body, controlled by the seven *chakra* centres, is similar to the Chinese meridian system and the location of its major acupoints. This is not just coincidence; there is historical evidence that the Hindu and Buddhist *chakra* system influenced Taoist and Confucian thinking when Buddhism spread into China via Tibet.

The *chakra* system is sometimes linked to the Western biomedical glandular system. The endocrine system, via its chemical messengers – the hormones that circulate in the blood – regulates the activities of our organs and tissues, and plays an important part in regulating our immune system and our reactions to stress. Connected to this is the lymphatic system, which is critical in maintaining our immune function. Each of the seven *chakras* is linked to a specific gland, and work on each *chakra* is thought to affect these glands in the physical body as well as affecting the emotional and mental functions connected to each *chakra*. So, for example, the second or sacral *chakra*; which is located behind the navel, is thought to correspond to the lymphatic system on the physical level and to self-empowerment and creativity on a higher level, while the fifth or throat *chakra* is linked to the thyroid and parathyroid glands in the physical body, and to communication or expression at a mental and emotional level.

In comparative terms, the endocrine system sends hormones around the body via the blood, which also circulates lymph, while in the *chakras*, energy is moved up through each one to achieve balance in both the physical and energetic bodies. If any of the *chakras* are not functioning properly, this will be reflected in the physical body through illness. Similarly, in Chi kung, the blood follows the *chi* and if the *chi* becomes blocked or stagnant, then the blood is also. Furthermore, organs start to suffer from *chi* deficiency. This might be compared to hormone deficiency on one level and a weakened immune system due to imbalance in the lymphatic system. The comparison between the different systems is not exact, but it provides a bridge between the physical and the energetic views.

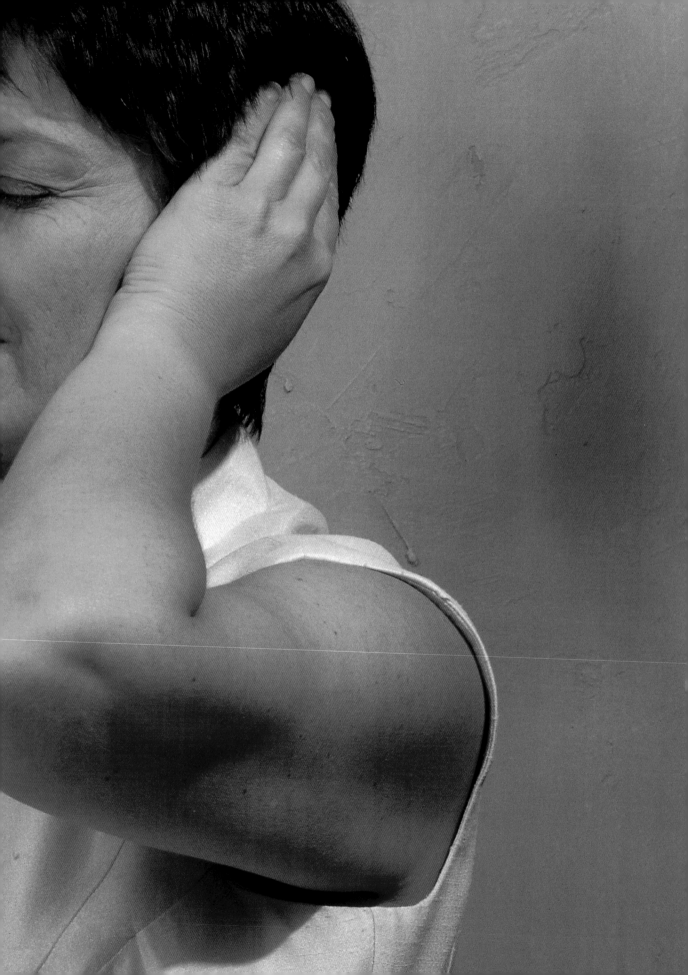

chi kung & stress

At the most basic level, Chi kung can be said to work by balancing the autonomic nervous system; when balanced, this results in improved functioning in all the other systems.

What causes problems in the autonomic nervous system? The answer is stress. Stress is now acknowledged to be the root cause of an ever-increasing number of health problems, both physical and mental. Twenty years ago few people had heard of stress as we understand the term today. The concept of psychosomatic factors and the influence of the emotions on our health were still in their infancy. Even ten years ago it was not generally accepted that stress is a major factor in physical ill-health, although there was a growing acknowledgment of its role and of the interdependence of mind and body. Understanding has grown rapidly since then. This is partly due to the growth in popularity of complementary medicine and the promotion of its ideas in the media, but also because the medical establishment has found the connection through its own studies. It is now not so unusual for medical practitioners to diagnose stress as the cause of illness, and they are also more likely to advise patients to use relaxation techniques to relieve their stress.

Reacting to stress is a natural function of the nervous system and we all need some stress in our lives or we wouldn't be motivated to do anything. However, we all react differently, which indicates that a strong mental factor is involved. For example, driving is enormously stressful for some people, while others can't get enough of it. For others, the sources of stress are not confined to daily activities such as work, relationships and finances; stress may also come from the fear of living in an increasingly violent society, from the fear of war, and from the fear of being slowly poisoned by the food we eat and the air we breathe in our environmentally polluted times.

Stress, it could be said, is fundamentally caused for most people by the feeling of not being in control. This takes us back to the idea of 'going with the flow' or, in Taoist thinking, of cultivating suppleness in our response to life. When we feel in harmony with our environment, we feel strong and able to cope. We will still have challenges or problems – these are essential to our growth – but when we are relaxed and able to bend like a tree in the wind, we are more capable of finding solutions that avoid the build-up of stress.

Chi kung, meditation techniques and autogenic training are all effective methods for controlling the autonomic nervous system and thereby relieving stress. This is because they all emphasize controlling the breath. When we encounter a stress factor we are aware of the change in our breathing as well as the increased heart rate, dry mouth and sweating caused by the surge of adrenaline in the sympathetic nervous system. I remember a time when I was under extreme stress at work and went through several months of not sleeping or eating properly. After a while I began to sense an unusual taste in my mouth, and intuitively I knew that the taste was that of adrenaline – the result of being in a constantly over-stressed state. I didn't know about relaxation techniques then, but if I had, perhaps I would not have left that particular job – a rather drastic method of stress relief.

Controlling your breathing by slowing it down and focusing your attention on it will then control all the other uncomfortable symptoms. However, as we are under stress on a regular basis, we also need to control its effects regularly. Of course there are different levels of stress, but we are now so used to living with constant stress at some level that we are less aware of it and we have become used to its effect on our bodies.

The nervous system helps us to sense what is going on everywhere in our bodies. In Chi kung, it is believed that the mind leads the *chi* around the body, but if we are unable to feel what is happening in parts of our body then we cannot lead the *chi* there. However, when we are relaxed, we enter a state of heightened awareness of our body. This is the effect of the parasympathetic nervous system which, as previously explained, counteracts the action of the sympathetic system. However, if we live in a constant state of stress, the parasympathetic system does not have a chance to work and our body stays in stress mode.

We have a tendency to think that relaxation means sitting down and watching television, or reading a book. But these activites are not really relaxing, as your mind is constantly engaged. Even taking part in some sports, while good for your body, requires strategic thinking that means you are not completely relaxed. Full relaxation is only achieved when the mind – which leads the body – is also relaxed in a meditative state. Chi kung is an extremely effective means of achieving that state. Research in China into the benefits of Chi kung shows that when the body is relaxed, the tension in the sympathetic nerves is reduced and the action of the parasympathetic nerves increases. This improves the coordination between the two systems so that the body remains in a relaxed, reflexive state. This is extremely important for both preventing and curing illness. In other words, when the two systems are in harmony it is easier for us to revert from an alert state to a relaxed state, whereas when the systems are unbalanced it is more difficult for us to become tranquil.

chi kung anatomy & natural body cycles

meridians

Having already looked at how Chi kung acts on the body from the perspective of Western anatomy and physiology, we must now consider it in terms of the energy anatomy. The meridian system (see right) is the foundation of the energy anatomy. It operates parallel to the physical body, and at the same time complements it. Like the *chakras*, the meridians are in energetic control of the denser physical body. The meridians conduct *chi*, and are the starting point for a never-ending cycle of events in the body, which run in the following sequence:

air (*chi*) – blood – cells – tissues – organs – functions – relationships – the Whole

In Chi kung, the mind leads *chi*, the *chi* leads the blood, which in turn feeds the cells that constitute the tissue, which in turn forms the organs. The organs carry out the functions, which are all related and together form the Whole.

The 12 major meridians are each related to a specific organ as well as to the senses and emotions and the whole system is joined to form a continuous circuit, which loops around three times through the main meridians.

chi kung points – the energy gates

The meridians all have acupoints and anyone who has received acupuncture treatment will be familiar with these. The points are near the surface of the body, where the energy passing through them can be affected by needles, by the hands, or by visualization. There are 670 acupoints on the meridians, but Chi kung requires you to learn only nine basic points. The location of these points is given in a table at the back of the book (see page 125) where I have listed both the Western name and its Chinese equivalent.

As you become more skilled in your practice of Chi kung you will become increasingly aware of these points, and in fact for most Chi kung exercises you will need to be aware of them since they are integral to the control of *chi*.

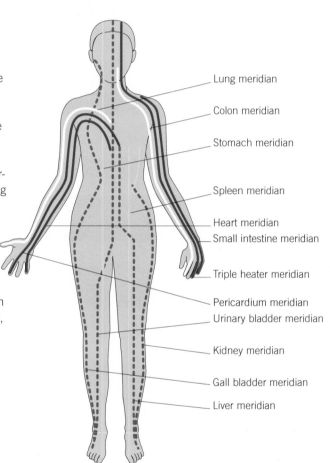

Lung meridian
Colon meridian
Stomach meridian
Spleen meridian
Heart meridian
Small intestine meridian
Triple heater meridian
Pericardium meridian
Urinary bladder meridian
Kidney meridian
Gall bladder meridian
Liver meridian

the 12 major meridians

the *dantian*

The body is divided into three energy centres, referred to as the lower, middle and upper *Dantian*, which are linked by the Governor and Conception channels of the meridian system. The lower *Dantian* is just below the navel and is where your power (not to be confused with *chi* energy) is stored. Most of the exercises in this book encourage you to focus on the lower *Dantian*, as it is the centre of your essence. The middle *Dantian*, just above the navel, is the centre of emotions and *chi*, while the upper *Dantian*, is concerned with our mental and spiritual aspects.

Before you can start to work with the two upper centres, you need to learn to control the lower centre in order to ground the *chi* energy. If you do not learn to do that first, you may experience various physical and emotional upsets associated with not being centered.

the three treasures

At an even more basic level than the meridians, acupoints and *Dantian*, there are the Three Treasures, which are considered to the foundations of our total composition. They are known as *jing*, *chi* and *shen*.

Jing – this is our inherited or genetic energy, and Chi kung has methods for tapping into this store. It is also our sexual energy, which needs to be preserved. Again, Chi kung has a number of methods for utilizing sexual energy for improving health as well as sexual experience.

Chi – this is the vital essence that we depend on for life. It has different forms within the body, such as *yuan chi*, *wei chi* and *ku chi*, and the foundation of a person's *chi* is the quality of their *jing*. This *chi* is the same as the *chi* energy referred to throughout the book, and is one of the three forms of energy recognized along with *jing* and *shen*.

Shen – this is our spirit or soul, which is fed by our *chi*.

The Three Treasures are hierarchical:, *jing* feeding *chi* and *chi* feeding *shen*. Chi kung cannot alter our innate genetic character but it can help us tap into it to help support and develop our *chi* (see page 26). As we develop our *chi*, our spirit is cultivated and so through Chi kung we can achieve better health and a new level of spiritual consciousness.

chi kung and biorhythms

According to Oriental anatomy and physiology, the functioning of the body follows natural cycles – the rhythms of nature. We recognize the effects of the lunar cycle on the tides and on our psyche, but our path around the sun also creates rhythms that affect us unconsciously. For example, are you aware that between 3am and 5am, the flow of *chi* peaks in your lungs? As it keeps up its constant flow around the body during the 24 hours of the day, *chi* peaks in each of the 12 major organs for two of those hours each day.

Heart   11am–1pm
Gall bladder   11pm–1am
Small intestine   1pm–3pm
Liver   1am–3am
Bladder   3pm–5pm
Lungs   3am–5am
Kidneys   5pm–7pm
Colon   5am–7am
Pericardium   7pm–9pm
Stomach   7am–9am
Triple heater   9pm–11pm
Spleen   9am–11am

Note: The Triple Heater is a body function rather than an organ. It refers to a function of *chi* that controls the balance of heat and moisture in three regions of the body: the head and chest, the solar plexus and the lower abdomen.

With each season *chi* also peaks in a pair of organs. In spring it is the gall bladder and liver; in summer, it is the small intestine and heart; in late summer, the stomach and spleen; in autumn, the colon and lungs; and in winter, the bladder and kidneys. In order to prevent illness, you should be aware of the effects of each season on the body and adapt your lifestyle accordingly. This includes making changes to dietary and sleeping habits, as well as ensuring that you are wearing the right type of clothing. Chinese medicine and Chi kung in particular place great emphasis on protecting the body from cold, particularly the back and kidney area. It is also important to note that although Chi kung should ideally be practised outdoors, it should not be practised when it is either cold or windy as this will disturb your *chi*. Similarly, you should keep your feet warm when practising, even indoors, therefore wearing socks or Chinese slippers is advisable.

chi kung & medical questions

One of the great strengths of Chi kung is that everyone can do it, whatever their level of fitness. Also, since Chi kung can be practised standing, sitting or lying down, it is highly suitable for people with a physical disability. However, as with any physical activity, there are guidelines for practising Chi kung, which apply to the fit as well as to those people with specific physical problems.

• Always do the warm-up routine to release muscle tension and stretch the soft tissues before starting the exercises. Although the exercises are not strenuous, you will not get the same benefits from them if you do not loosen the body up a little beforehand. Ill health is due to stagnation and this may make static postures impossible. If static postures are painful, do not practise them in the early stages.

• Do not practise on an empty stomach or after a heavy meal. Make sure you always keep your feet warm by wearing socks or slippers.

• During pregnancy certain precautions should be taken and some exercises avoided. For example, you should avoid exercises that move the internal organs. You should also focus your attention above the area of the uterus. Many exercises ask you to bring energy down into the navel area – if you are pregnant, keep the energy higher up.

• The precautions that apply to pregnancy apply to some extent to menstruating women, because Chi kung exercises that involve bringing energy down into the navel and pelvic area will increase the flow of blood. Also, if you are feeling tired or if you are low emotionally, it might be better to refrain from practice for a day or two, or simply do only the relaxation routine.

• People with mental health problems should avoid those aspects of Chi kung that involve too much mental concentration, such as emptying or clearing the mind. Focus instead on using Chi kung for relaxation and for centring and earthing energy.

• If you have a specific health problem, and particularly if you are under the supervision of a doctor, you should consult him or her before beginning to practise Chi kung.

the healing smile

This exercise can be done as part of your daily routine or before you get up in the morning. It is a very simple method of checking the condition of your body and thanking it for working so efficiently. You can do the exercise standing, sitting or lying down.

Step 1
Relax your body and place your hands over your navel. Close your eyes and focus your attention on your body. If your mind starts to wander, just bring your attention back to the body. Now think of something that makes you smile gently, and feel the energy of your smile grow.

Step 2
In Chi kung, energy follows the mind, so with your mind direct the energy of your smile to your internal organs. Begin with your heart. Send the smile to your heart and see how your heart feels. Hold the energy there for as long as you want and thank your heart for its work. Now direct the energy to your lungs, and follow the same process as for your heart. From your lungs, move to your liver, then to your kidneys, then to your spleen, each time repeating the process.

Step 3
Now, relax your smile and lead the energy from all your organs down to your navel, gathering it together at the *Dantian*, the storehouse of your energy.

Focus your attention at the navel and experience the energy collected there. Make a mental note of how at peace your body feels now, and finish the exercise by slowly opening your eyes and relaxing your hands. You can then rub your palms together and wipe them over your face and head to make you feel alert again.

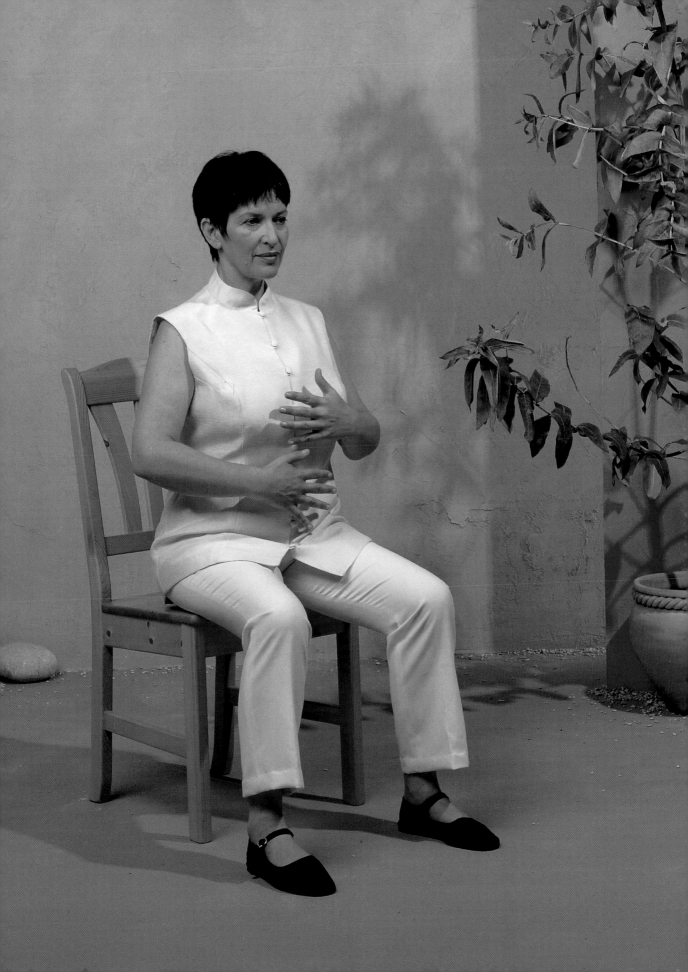

an everyday routine

Our bodies are full of energy, but because of the everyday stresses of living this energy becomes blocked inside us. We begin life full of vitality, but from the moment of birth we are in constant movement. When our bodies are resting, our minds are moving – even as we sleep. As our bodies age, they react to this by accumulating tension in the muscles and nerves. This weakens our internal organs and immune system, so that by the end of our lives we find that the vitality we had at birth has slipped away. If we knew how to relax fully – and that means relaxing the mind as well as the body – we would be able to draw on that innate vitality, the *chi*, that is with us from birth.

Practising Chi kung develops internal strength and energy. It also teaches us to relax our entire system and calm our minds so that we can remove our internal energy blocks. A few minutes' practice daily will help you to reclaim the vitality that is naturally yours.

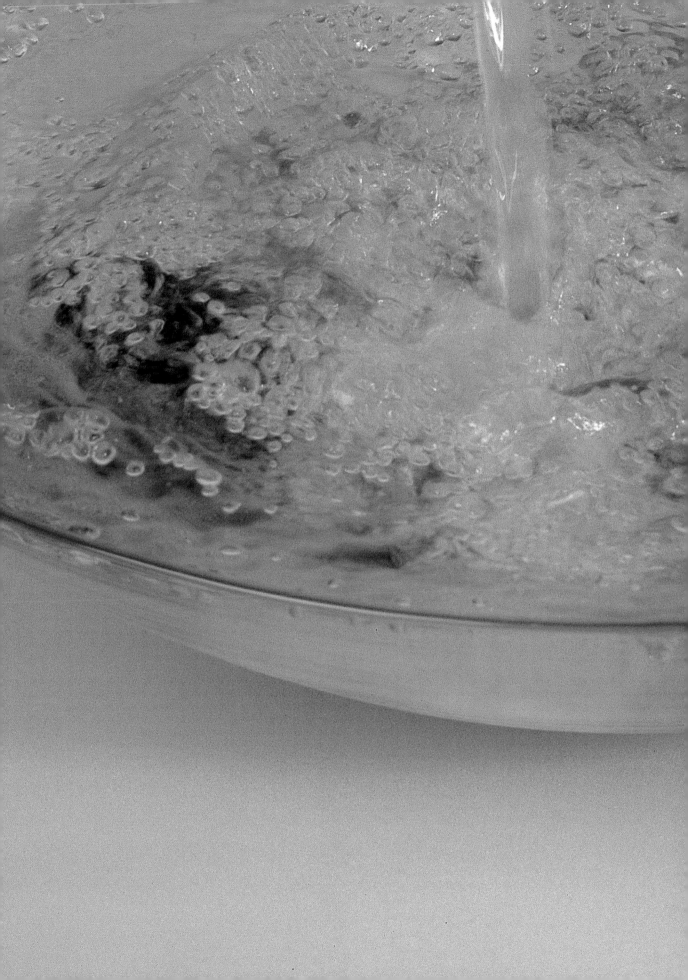

the benefits of regular practice

The effects of Chi kung build up over time. Some classes may be held weekly for a short period of eight to ten weeks, while others may be ongoing on a regular basis. You will feel the benefits during and immediately after the class, but your body needs to relearn how to relax and that means regularly teaching it, by practising between classes, and continuing your practice once the series of lessons has ended. If you don't, your body will simply revert to its old habits.

Unfortunately most of us have such busy lives we find it hard to make time to look after ourselves. However, even if you practise for 15 minutes every day you will be building up long-term benefits – and don't give up because these benefits aren't immediately noticeable. Our bodies have been accumulating the effects of stress since birth, so they are not likely to show a major improvement within a few weeks. If you can't manage to practise Chi Kung every day to begin with, start with two or three times a week. Also, remember that while you are travelling to work you can practise focusing on the breath, or even the healing smile exercise.

There are of course ideal conditions in which to practise Chi kung. As mentioned previously, practising in a group increases your experience of *chi* energy, which is why every morning parks in China are filled with people doing Chi kung. But most of us must be content with practising alone on a daily basis. If the weather is good, try to practise outdoors, as more *chi* is available to you there, especially where there are trees or other greenery as they generate a lot of energy. But do not exercise outdoors if it is raining, cold or windy. Also, wear comfortable clothes that allow free body movement. Don't strain your body – you won't achieve the benefits of Chi kung any faster by pushing yourself beyond your limits, or by practising for long periods of time. Always do the warm-ups first and finish your session by rubbing your hands together, shaking your arms and legs and ensuring that you feel grounded. Finally, do not practise if you are unwell, overtired or emotionally upset, as this will distract you from your practice.

Finally, you might find, as I do, that playing relaxing music with a gentle rhythm will help you to create more flowing body movements in both the warm-up exercises and the Chi kung postures. This is very important, because Chi kung is all about flow and rhythms, with softly rounded limb movements. Listening to the circular progressions of melody while exercising will heighten your awareness of those qualities.

what happens during chi kung?

The long-term effects on the mind and body of practising Chi kung follow a sequence which has the following effects:

Cleanses
You begin by ridding your body of any pathogenic or harmful *chi*, by using exhalation of the breath, shaking it from your body and visualizing it leaving.

Generates
You learn to focus your attention on the energy in your lower *Dantian* or navel area. This is where energy enters your body and is the point to which you should move energy mentally.

Increases
You increase your *chi* by building and preserving it in your body. You also increase your ability to draw *chi* from external sources such as trees and sunlight.

Accumulates
You develop the ability to hold larger amounts of *chi* within your body.

Refines
Once you have learnt how to build up and control your *chi*, you then learn how to refine it. This principally means refining your emotions so that they

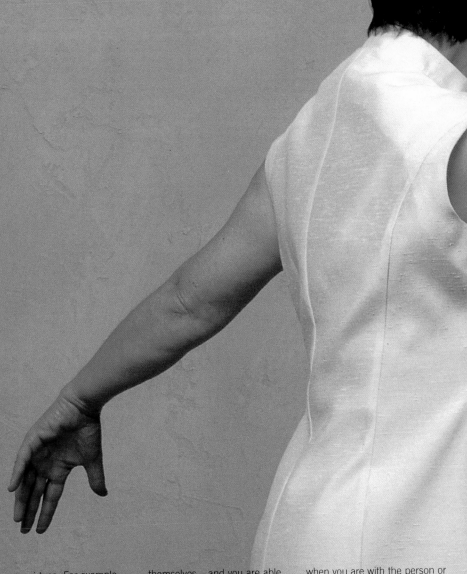

become virtues. For example, anger (from the liver and gall bladder) becomes kindness, or fear (kidneys and bladder) becomes gentleness.

Circulates

Your refined *chi* is then circulated through the entire meridian system and out into the etheric body or aura field. You will now be able to sense where energy is blocked and be able to remove the blockage by using your mind.

Stores

At this stage you can store the refined energy at the deepest levels of your body – in the cells

themselves – and you are able to absorb even more energy from outside.

Preserves

This means preserving your own *chi* and being able to protect yourself within your own energy field so that negative influences, either from the environment or from other people, will not disturb your *chi*.

Discharges

When you have got to this final stage you will have built up your *chi* sufficiently to be able to pass it on to others in order to give them healing. This can be done

when you are with the person or over long distances; there are many amazing stories about the ability of Chi kung masters to transmit *chi* in this way.

It takes time – years not months – of regular practice to progress from cleansing yourself of harmful *chi* and learning how to increase it in your physical body, to being able to transmit it to others. Progress often seems to happen spontaneously in Chi kung, therefore consciously pushing yourself to achieve the higher levels may actively work against improving your physical health and your spiritual growth.

essential warm-ups

You should always take time to do the warm-up routine. It is advisable with most sports to warm up the muscles and loosen the joints before fully exerting yourself, otherwise you risk beginning your exercises with cold muscles and stiff joints, which can lead to problems with them rather than help them. Although Chi kung exercises are not particularly strenuous – compared to an aerobic workout, for example – you are moving energy around the body and this will be easier if the body has already been loosened up to allow the energy to flow more easily.

You should also ensure that you clear yourself of harmful *chi* before bringing fresh *chi* into the body. If you do not, it is a bit like cleaning a room by sweeping the dirt under the carpet. You can start to clear away harmful *chi* during the warm-ups by firmly brushing it off your arms and by shaking it off your hands and feet. See it leave your body and disintegrate. When you start the Chi kung exercises, the Shower of Light (page 52) will cleanse bad *chi* from the aura field around your body. The aura is a subtle energy field surrounding the body and extending beyond it for about 10–15 cm (4–6 in). It is thought to reflect the emotional and physical state of each one of us, although it can only be seen by relatively few people.

The warming-up sequence should be done for a minimum of five minutes, but the length of time you spend on each part of it is a matter of individual choice.

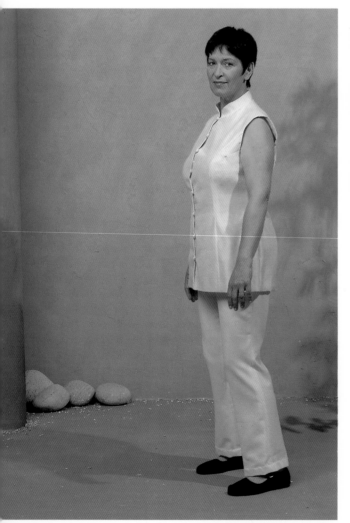

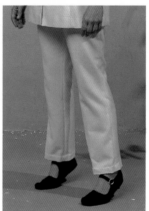

bouncing on your feet

Step 1
Start by standing with your feet placed shoulder-width apart and your arms relaxed.

Step 2
Bounce up and down on your feet, raising your heel slightly off the floor but keeping the ball of your foot firmly on it. If you want, you can swing your arms gently forwards and backwards as this will add momentum to your rhythm, but keep your rhythm steady rather than too energetic. This exercise allows your internal organs to massage each other, so you are warming them up as well as your muscles and joints.

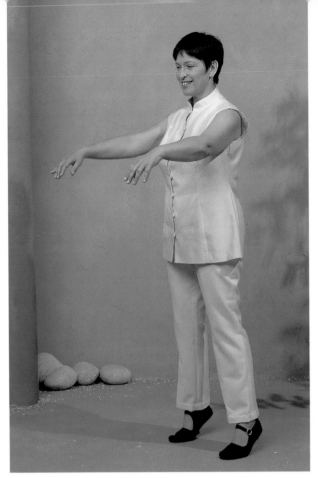

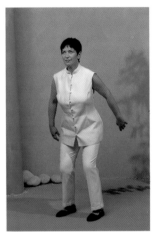

swinging arms forwards and backwards

Step 1

Stop bouncing and start to swing
your arms more energetically
forwards and backwards, rising
on your toes and inhaling as you
bring your arms up and exhaling
as you swing your arms down
behind you.

Step 2

When exhaling on the backward
swing, I find it helps to really
blow your breath out through
your lips so that you get the
sense of ridding yourself of stale
air and toxins in your lungs.

You can also do a variation
of this exercise with a partner.
One person stands still while
the other stands on one side of
them and swings the other
person's arm for them, pushing
it back and forth using their
hands. They then change to
the other side.

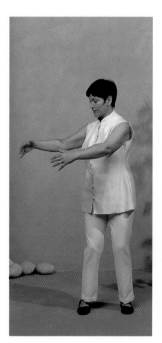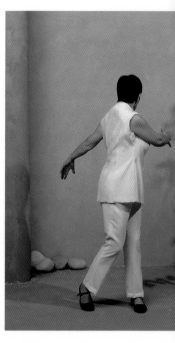

swinging arms from side to side

Step 1
Keeping the same rhythm, swing your arms from left to right across the front of your body. As you do this, your waist and hips will naturally want to move with each swing. Now as you swing your arms you can start moving from one foot to the other.

Step 2
When you swing your arms to the left, keep your weight on your left foot and raise the heel of your right foot off the ground. When you swing to the right, your weight will be on your right foot and your left foot will naturally rise.

swinging arms around the body

Step 1
Move from the last exercise into this, keeping your weight moving from one foot to the other as before. Swing your arms to the left, allowing your right hand to touch your waist; at the same time your left arm will wrap around your back, so the back of your hand touches the right-hand side of your back. When swinging to the right, your left hand will touch your right waist and your right hand will swing around to touch the left side of your back.

Step 2
Once you have established your rhythm, turn your head to the left, looking over your left shoulder as you swing your arms to the left, then turn it to the right, looking over your right shoulder as you swing your arms to the right. Remember to keep your breathing in rhythm with your body movements.

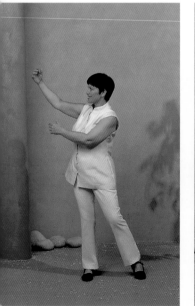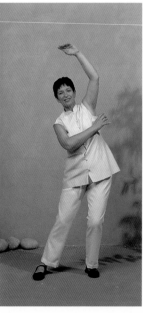

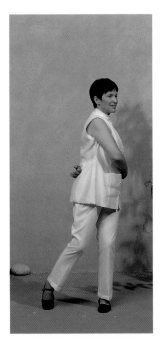

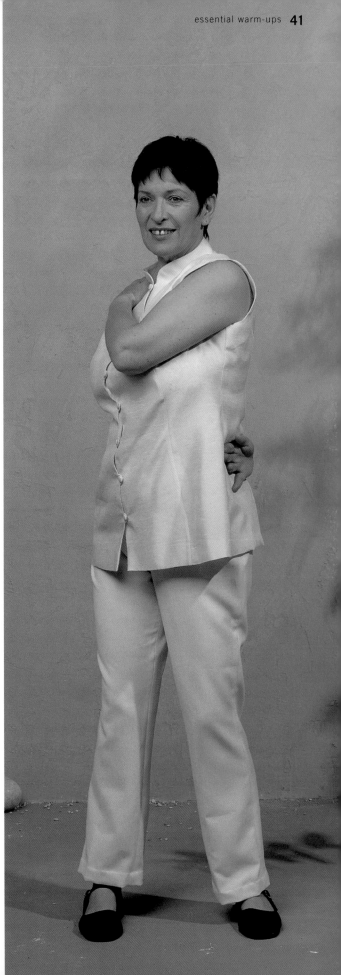

swinging arms and tapping the body

Step 1

Continue with the same movements as in the previous exercise, but now as you swing your arms across to the left, let your right hand hit the side of your left hip and your left hand hit the top of your right buttock. Repeat this, swinging to the right. Keeping your rhythm, start to move up your body, hitting yourself at the waist, front and back. Do this several times.

Step 2

Then, swinging right, hit your right shoulder with your left hand, while your right hand hits the back of your waist on your left side. Do this several times, then move down to your hips again and repeat the sequence, moving up and down your body.

Repeat on the opposite side; still keeping your arms and body in the swinging rhythm, hit your arms, thighs or any part of your body that you feel needs it. This exercise activates your acupoints, so your body will let you know which ones need more stimulation.

knocking at the door of life

You can enhance the effects of
the last exercise by finishing it
with a Chi kung action called
'Knocking at the Door of Life'.
This exercise activates the two
main energy 'gates' on the
Governor and Conception channels. These are located at the
level of the navel in the front,
and on the back at the point in
your lumbar region called the
Mingmen or Door of Life. This
is important because it is
connected to your kidneys,
where your genetic or ancestral
chi energy is stored. Let each of
your hands form a loose fist and
now, when you swing your arms
to the left, hit both these points
with your fists. Continue to twist
your body and head in each
direction, as in the previous
exercise.

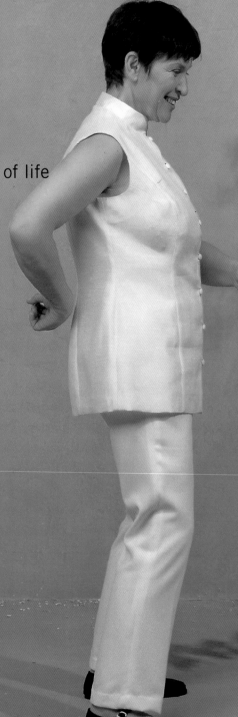

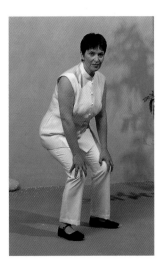

warming up knees

We don't give our knees much attention and this exercise will help to loosen them up. Standing with your feet slightly apart, bend your knees and lean forward so that your fingers can just touch them, but keep your head up and look ahead. Keeping your fingers there, rotate both knees together several times to the left. Do the same number of rotations, this time to the right.

The position of the knees is important in Chi kung exercises, as keeping them slightly bent helps the energy to flow.

releasing stagnant *chi*

At this point you can get rid of the accumulated *chi* that causes illness. Imagine letting go of your emotional blockages, too.

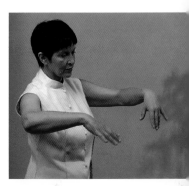

Step 1
Do this by first of all shaking your hands, allowing your wrists to go limp. Shake your hands hard from side to side.

Step 2
Now lift one foot and shake it vigorously, then the other. If you have any balance problems, hold on to the back of a chair while shaking your feet.

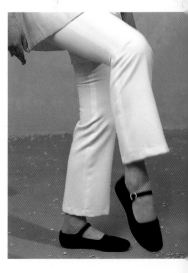

Step 3
You can also make firm sweeping movements down your arms, exhaling loudly with each downward stroke, as if you were brushing off dirt.

You can use this particular movement before starting the Meridian Massage (see page 44). Remember to visualize the stagnant *chi* leaving your body while doing all of these movements. Also, every out-breath is releasing toxins from the body as you exhale carbon dioxide, to be replaced by fresh oxygen as you breathe in.

Now you are ready to move into the next exercise, the Meridian Massage, which will open up the meridian channels in the upper body, particularly those relating to the heart and lungs and general circulation.

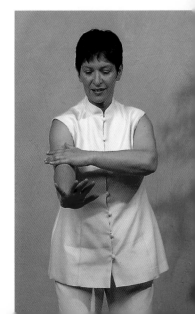

meridian massage

This exercise helps to open up the major meridians in the upper body and follows on naturally from the movements for cleansing blocked *chi* from the channels. Cleanse blocked *chi* by brushing down the arms and legs, and anywhere else on the body you can easily reach, as if you were brushing dirt off your clothes with your hands. Make sure that your strokes are long, definite and rhythmic. It may help if you imagine ridding yourself of emotional problems and yesterday's arguments and mistakes.

The Meridian Massage uses the same rhythmic movement – swaying from left to right – as the warm-up exercises, and doing it to music will help you to establish a flowing rhythm. Beginners and people with shoulder problems should not raise their arms too high to begin with. Although the instructions are given in steps, this exercise should be performed as one continuous and flowing movement.

Begin by standing with your right foot on the floor and the heel of your left foot raised.

When doing this exercise, you move your body weight from one foot to the other, putting your weight on your right foot when stroking your right arm while raising the heel of your left foot off the floor, and vice versa. It may help you to practise this movement before beginning the Meridian Massage, swinging both your arms from side to side at the same time as moving your body, so that you become familiar with what your lower body should be doing before you add in the massage movements.

Once you have mastered

this, you will build up a flowing rhythm, combining stroking movements up and down your arms at the same time as moving your body from side to side. Remember your breathing and you will find that it, too, falls in with your natural rhythm. Do the Meridian Massage for as long as it feels right for you. Six repetitions of the sequence are the minimum required, eventually building up to 36 repetitions.

If you find this exercise difficult to begin with, simply stroke down the left arm as it swings across the body, then

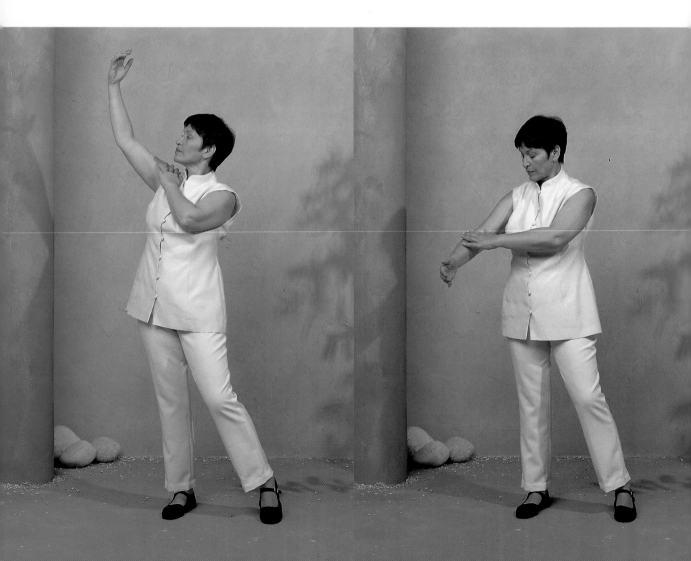

rubbing hands and gathering energy

stroke down the right arm as you swing it across. Repeat this motion as before.

Step 1
Start with your left hand on your right shoulder and your right arm raised.

Step 2
Stroke down the outside of your right arm as you swing the arm across your body.

Step 3
When your left hand reaches the fingertips, your right hand then

strokes up the inside of your left arm to the shoulder as you bring your left arm above your head.

Step 4
When your right hand reaches your left shoulder, sweep it down the outside of your left arm to the fingertips, swinging the arm down at the same time. Now the left hand strokes up the inside of the right arm and when it reaches the shoulder again, it sweeps down the outside of the right arm. The right hand then strokes up the inside of the left arm, repeating the sequence.

Having loosened and relaxed your body, stimulated your energy flow and got rid of the stagnant *chi*, you can finish off your warm-ups by rubbing the palms of your hands together in a circular motion. This gathers the good *chi* you have built up in your warm-up session in your hands, and you can then rub your hands over your face as if you were washing it. This stimulates the flow of *chi* through your facial skin, improving your skin tone and general appearance. When you practise Chi kung, the *chi* energy flows

through five progressive levels: skin, flesh, meridians, bones and internal organs. You are therefore likely to see the first benefits of Chi kung in the appearance of your skin.

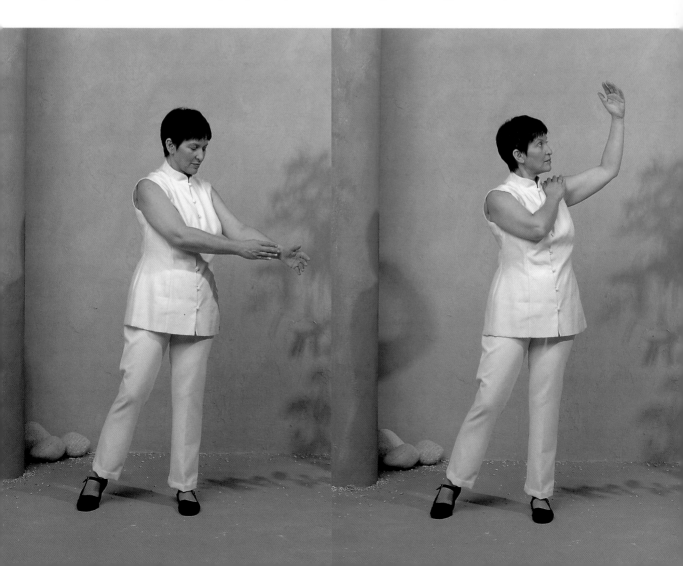

the chi kung posture

Poor posture is increasingly common. Our idea of relaxing the tension in our bodies is to slump down into a soft sofa where we keep our spines bent for hours on end. At work, many people sit at desks, shoulders hunched and rounded. Over time our muscles become used to these postures, and we find that we cannot regain the natural, straight-backed posture we had as children.

Posture, or simply learning to stand, sit or lie correctly, is an important element of Chi kung, because when your body is correctly aligned, you are drawing energy from the earth and accelerating its flow through your body. The two points you need to be most aware of are *Huiyin*, which lies at the perineum, in front of the anus, and *Baihui*, at the crown of your head (see right). These two need to be in alignment for *chi* to flow unimpeded through the skeleton and spine.

Both the sitting and the standing postures (below and right) are the basic positions for all Chi kung practice, and in themselves are powerful ways of unlocking your internal energy. Although they appear simple, and with practice are indeed simple, it may take some time before you feel completely comfortable in these positions.

Certainly, at first, you may find it difficult to hold these postures for long. If you do feel tension or discomfort anywhere, shake your arms and legs and then resume the posture. With practice you will learn to relax completely and you will be able to stand still for increasingly long periods. Follow the warm-up routine given earlier (see pages 38–45), which will loosen your spine and with improved body awareness and balance you will find these basic Chi kung postures easier to assume.

sitting posture

Sit upright with your bottom on the edge of the chair and your knees and feet shoulder-width apart. Relax your eyes and look straight ahead. Place the backs of your hands on your knees and keep your fingers spread. Lengthen the spine and open the energy gates (see the standing posture, opposite). Then breathe in and drop your shoulders while also drawing the chin slightly inwards.

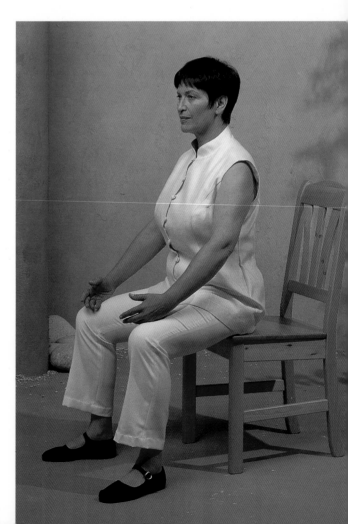

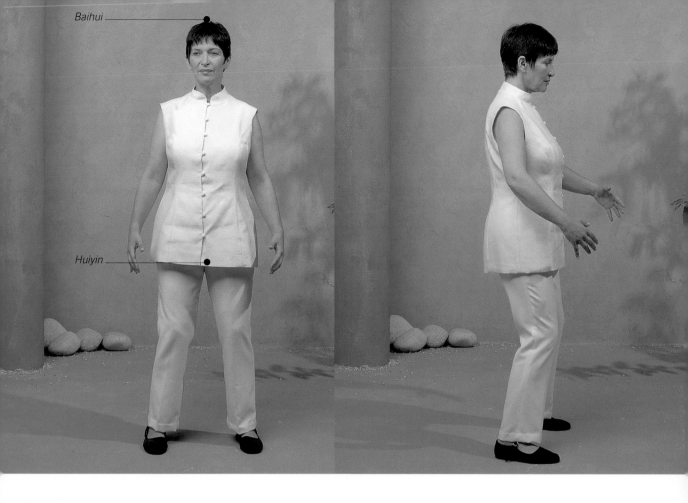

Baihui

Huiyin

standing posture: standing like a tree

Stand naturally with your feet together, then move your right foot out to shoulder distance from the left leg. Your feet should face straight forward and the knees should be slightly bent as though you were perching on a high stool – the pelvis will tilt up naturally as you do this. Your head should be upright, your face and eyelids relaxed, and your arms hanging naturally at the sides of the body. Think about your spine and feel it lengthen as you keep your weight and your centre of gravity in your lower legs.

Take a deep breath. When you exhale you will find that your shoulders will naturally lower and relax as if they are growing away from your ears. You should feel as if you are suspended from a point on the crown of

your head and the rest of your body is supported in air, with no tension anywhere.

As you inhale, you can then lengthen your spine and think about the four energy gates located at the *Huiyin* and *Baihui* points, and between the shoulder blades and at the base of the spine. Imagine that your armpits, your hands and the areas behind and between your knees are supported by balloons that make you feel soft and buoyant.

If you are not feeling well enough to stand, you can do this exercise sitting down. Choose a chair that is not too low so that you can keep your legs at right angles to your body with the knees not too bent, and your feet flat on the floor without straining.

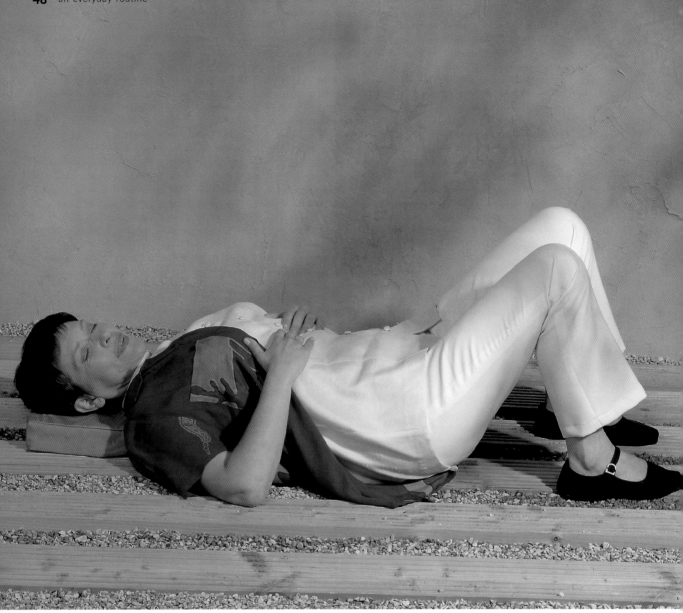

breathing technique

When practising the breathing technique, you might find it useful at first to place both hands on your abdomen, or one on your chest, so that you can feel the movement of your breath. You can practise this using the standing, sitting or lying (see above) Chi kung postures. The technique refers to nasal breathing, but people with blocked sinuses or similar conditions can breathe through the mouth.

Step 1

Begin by exhaling through your nose. At the end of the out-breath, tighten your stomach muscles and flatten your abdomen slightly. You will feel your diaphragm muscle push up as you do this, squeezing the air up and out of you. Push as much air out as you can without unnaturally forcing it, until you feel your lungs are empty. Now you have got rid of the stale air in your lungs you can take in clean air.

Step 2

Relaxing the stomach muscles, you will breathe in naturally and bring the air down into the abdomen so that it swells up under your hands like a balloon. Again, don't force this or you will create tension which will destroy the effect. Once your abdomen feels full of air, exhale again. Repeat until you feel familiar with the technique.

If you practise this technique regularly, you will find that you start to use this form of

breathing all the time without having to make yourself do it consciously. Then you will have returned to the way you breathed when you were first born. At first do not practise controlled breathing for more than three breaths at a time.

chi kung & breathing

Air is a primary source of energy for all of us and takes precedence over food, which is our other main energy source. At birth, the baby's first breath is also the first time that it draws energy into its body that has not come through the mother. Breathing is one of our body's automatic functions and we are usually unaware of it unless there is a problem. Nor do we think about the effect that breathing has on our other body systems – breathing is simply something that we do until we die.

Both your mental state and the state of your nervous system have a profound effect on your breathing and vice versa. When you are distressed or anxious, your chest area tends to tighten, your breathing becomes shallower and faster, and your heartbeat also quickens. Because your respiration is shallow you are not taking in enough oxygen; consequently you breathe faster to take in more, and so a cycle builds up which can result in hyperventilation accompanied by dizziness and fainting.

When we are in this state, we are convinced in our minds that we need to inhale more air, when in fact we actually need to exhale more. If you ask an asthmatic about their experiences during an attack, they will usually tell you that they feel they can't breathe in enough air, whereas medical research shows that the real problem is that they can't breathe enough air out. This is why in the Chi kung technique the emphasis is on the out-breath. It is exhalation that allows the body to relax, and if you exhale fully, your inward breath will automatically be fuller.

Just as anxiety states affect breathing, heart rate and digestion, they also affect your body's ability to circulate *chi* smoothly and to draw more *chi* into your system. By slowing down your breathing, or focusing your awareness on the breath as in some meditation techniques, you can reverse this situation; slow down your breathing and the heart rate also falls. The voluntary muscles also lose some of their tension as they receive more oxygen.

The ideal way to breathe is slowly and deeply, using the diaphragm muscle and abdomen, not the chest as most adults do. However, beginners, and anyone with breathing difficulties practising Chi kung, should not try to force changes in their breathing, or worry unduly about achieving slow, deep breaths. As your practice develops you can monitor the change yourself. The average person takes 16 breaths per minute, whereas after practising Chi kung for some time that can be reduced to five or less.

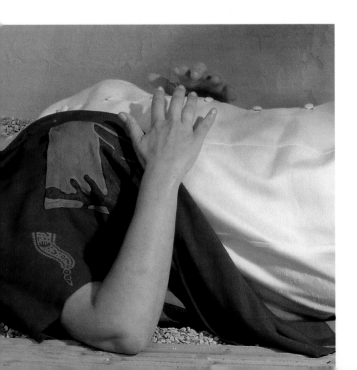

eight basic exercises

This series of eight everyday exercises is aimed primarily at improving your health. You do not need to do the entire sequence of exercises every time – you can start with just two or three instead. It is far better to spend your time learning and memorizing each exercise properly rather than trying to rush through them all. Some teachers say that beginners should start by practising for 15 minutes and gradually build up to 30-minute sessions or longer, and I think this is sound advice. If you don't have 15 minutes to spare, do what you can. Remember to do your warm-ups

and clearing of blocked *chi* energy (see pages 38–43) before starting these basic Chi kung exercises.

If you feel uncomfortable when doing the exercises, or you feel your centre of gravity has moved from being in front of you, you can move out of the Chi kung posture between each exercise, particularly if you are just beginning. It is better to move after every exercise, shaking your hands and feet a little, and then resume the standing position so that you feel entirely comfortable in it; then you can refocus on the *Baihui* and *Huiyin* points being properly aligned.

opening and closing the *chi*

The important thing with this exercise is focusing on the feelings of resistance when pushing down and pulling up. When pushing downwards, I have suggested imagining pushing a stick into the ground, but you could also imagine pushing a swimming float under the water, or you can find your own image which suggests to you that type of physical resistance. Similarly, when pulling your hands back up, visualize the backs of your hands having to pull away from the floor, using whatever image works best for you.

Step 1
Assume the standing posture (see pages 47). Relax your body by exhaling and allowing your shoulders to drop and aligning your *Baihui* point on the crown of your head with your *Huiyin* point at your perineum. Place the tip of your tongue against your hard palate, just behind your teeth. This is an important aid in helping *chi* energy to circulate in a complete circuit around the body, as it is part of

the alignment of *Baihui* and *Huiyin* – you should do it during all the Chi kung exercises in this book. Also, be aware of the kidney points or *Yongquan* on the soles of your feet – your Bubbling Springs – where the earth energy enters and where you connect with the earth. Inhaling, bring your arms in front of your body, palms up.

Step 2
Raise your arms to just below chest height. Your fingertips

should not touch but should point towards one other. Your hands should be loosely flexed with the fingers open.

Step 3
Rotate your arms inwards so that your palms are now facing downwards.

Step 4
Exhaling, press your hands down slowly as if you were pushing a stick into the ground. As you push downwards, allow

your body to bend down a little with the movement. Keep pushing down until your hands reach the navel area.

Continue by turning your palms over to face upwards and slowly bring them back up to chest height. Imagine that a rubber band is trying to pull your hands back down – feel the resistance. When you bring your hands back up, remember to keep your knees slightly bent. Repeat the whole sequence 4–6 times.

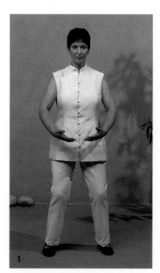

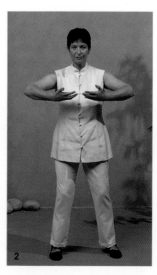

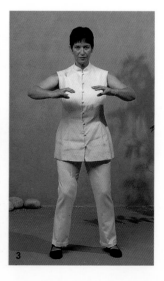

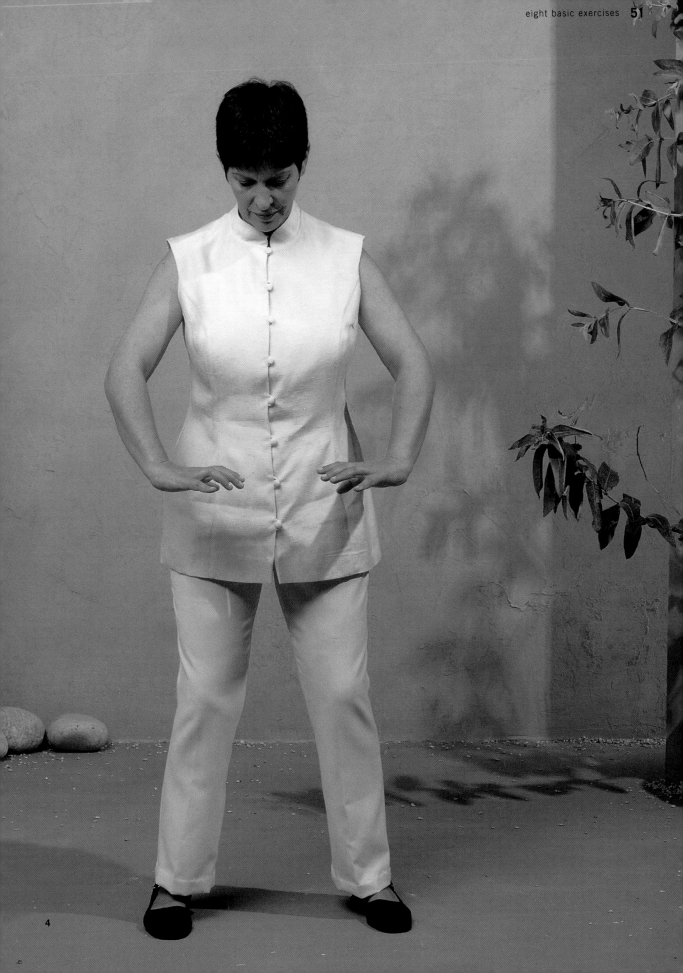

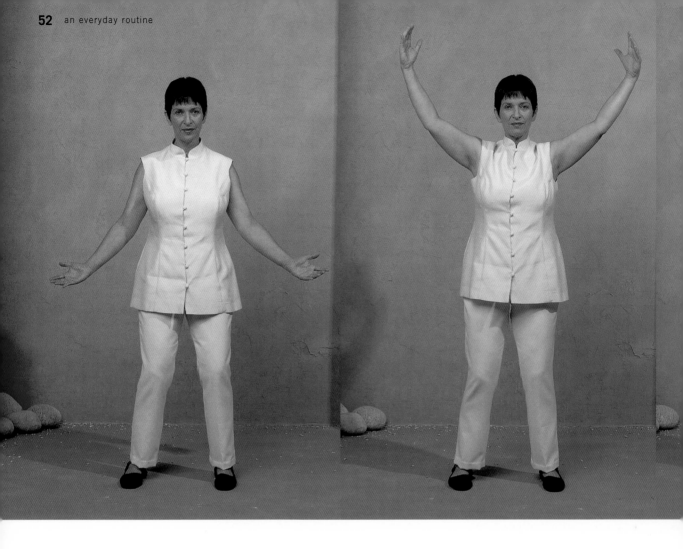

the shower of light

This is a wonderful exercise for drawing in fresh *chi* to energize you and for cleansing harmful *chi* from the energy field that surrounds you. It is a way of washing your body with energy rather than water, so visualize yourself standing in a shower.

Step 1
Take up the standing posture and ensure that your whole body is relaxed. With your arms at your sides, turn your palms to face outwards and upwards. Breathing in, slowly start to raise your arms up on both sides.

Step 2
Continue raising your arms, remembering not to straighten them out at any point but keep them relaxed and slightly rounded in shape (in Chi kung exercises the body never makes straight lines or sharp angles since this impedes the flow of *chi*). If you can, do Steps 1 and 2 whilst inhaling only, as it will be easier for you to hold on to the energy you have absorbed into your hands. However, if you need to exhale when your hands reach above your head, it is better to do that than hold your breath. Instead, use your mind to retain the energy.

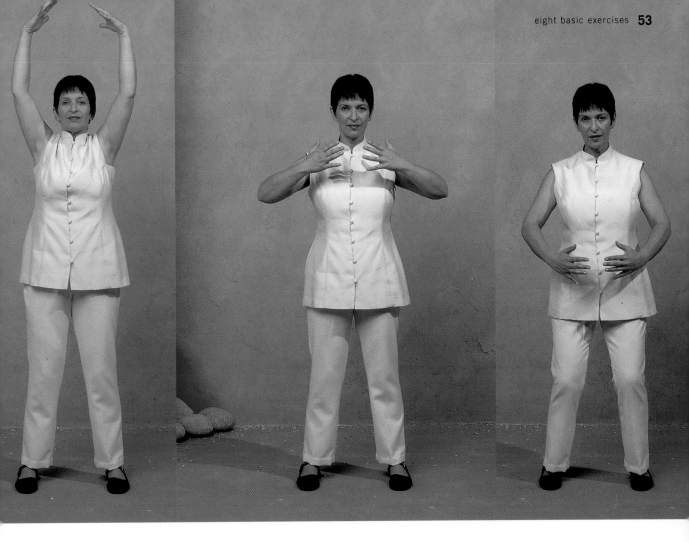

Step 3

When your arms are above your head, imagine fresh *chi* energy from the sky filling your palms. Visualize your palms as sponges soaking up the energy. Use your mind to hold the energy there.

Step 4

As you exhale, slowly bring your hands, palms still facing inwards, down over the top of your head, in front of your face.

Step 5

Continue bringing your arms down the front of your body until they reach your navel. As you do this, visualize the energy flowing down from the top of your head, down your front, your back and your sides, clearing out the harmful energy and replacing it with clean, fresh *chi*. Now bring your hands out to the sides again and repeat the sequence. Repeat this 4–6 times.

the eagle

For most Chi kung exercises you usually keep the eyelids relaxed to the point where they are nearly closed. Certainly this helps with learning to sense the energy and to focus on visualization without distraction. However, this can cause difficulty in an exercise which requires balancing on the balls of your feet and your toes. I have found that the best solution to the problem of keeping your balance is to keep your eyes open and look straight ahead. You will also perform the exercise more easily when your body

is very relaxed, so don't make it the first one in your routine.

The Eagle is an excellent exercise for improving your immune system. If you do not always include it in your Chi kung session, then it would be beneficial to include it in your routine at times of seasonal change when people are more prone to colds and 'flu, or when you hear that any type of viral infection is in the community.

Step 1

Start by assuming the correct standing posture, ensuring that

you feel balanced with your centre of gravity in front of you. Bring your hands, palms facing inwards and your fingers spread open, in front of your body, without having them touch each other. Remember always to maintain the feeling of roundness in your arms.

Step 2

Now, slowly draw your hands out to your sides and at the same time start to pull your arms towards your back. Your palms should now be facing the front with your thumbs uppermost.

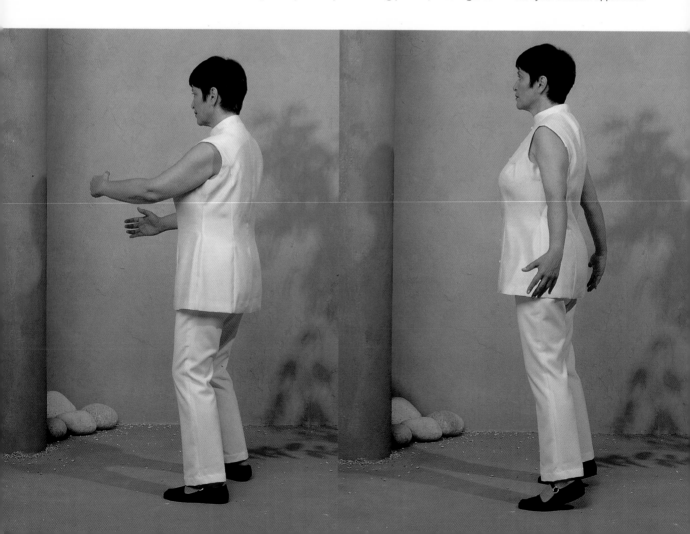

Step 3

Looking straight ahead, pull your arms back further until they are at a 45-degree angle from your back and shoulders. Your arms should still be kept slightly rounded, but you should feel that your outer arm is hard and resistant to pressure. This is similar to the experience of resistance in the first exercise (see page 50). While doing this keep your back straight and your chin drawn backwards. As you pull your arms into this position, lift your heels off the ground and balance on your

toes. Now visualize that you are a great eagle flying through the air. Your arms are your wings and the sun is warming them. Hold the position for a few seconds.

Step 4

Now bring your arms down to the starting position and at the same time place your heels back on the ground. While you are doing this exercise, breathe deeply but naturally. Repeat the sequence 4–6 times.

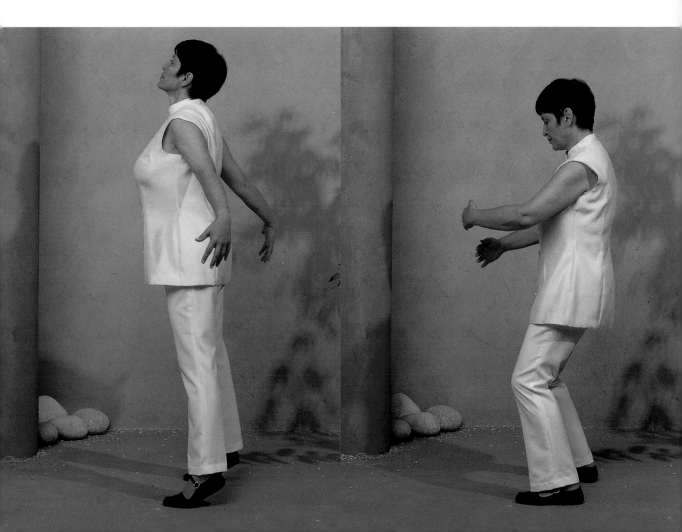

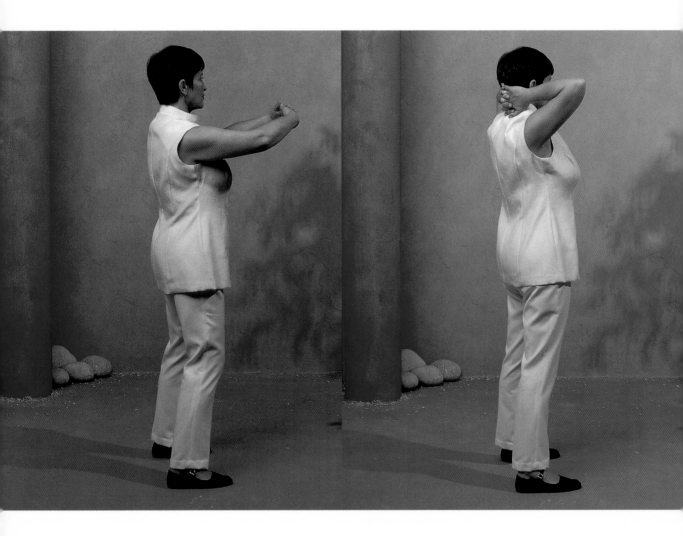

the bow

This exercise is beneficial for the bladder system and is also very useful for desk-bound workers, especially those who sit in front of computers for long periods of time. It is a simple exercise, but care should be taken not to force your arms any further back than is comfortable. With practice the muscles will keep opening up more, but don't try to force them.

Step 1

In the standing posture, bring your hands up to chest height and interlock your fingers.

Step 2

Now raise your interlocked hands over your head and place them over your occipital bone at the base of your skull, as if making a cradle for your head. In this position your elbows will be pointing out to the side.

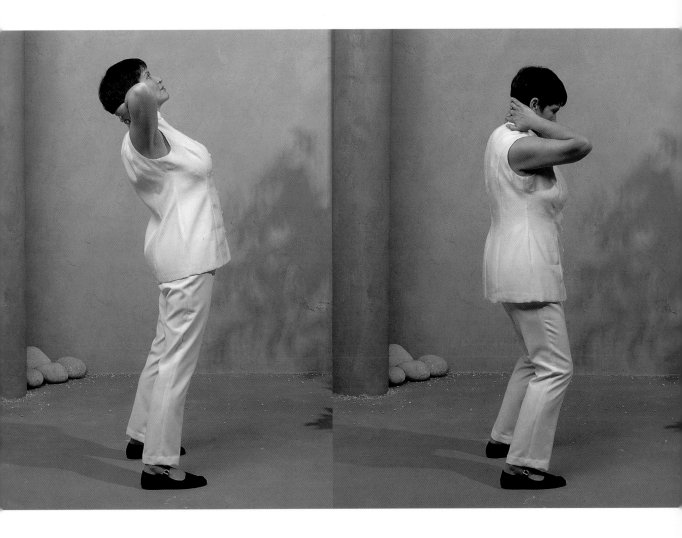

Step 3

Breathing in, push your head back against your hands and, as you do so, pull your elbows back and out to the side as far as you are comfortably able. You will feel your body start to arch back as you do this, and your chest and abdomen muscles will be pulled upwards and outwards.

Step 4

Exhaling, bring your elbows forwards again, but keep your hands behind your head. Allow the action to pull your head down as you breathe out. I find it helps to exhale fully at the end of the movement so that I feel the release. Repeat the sequence 4–6 times.

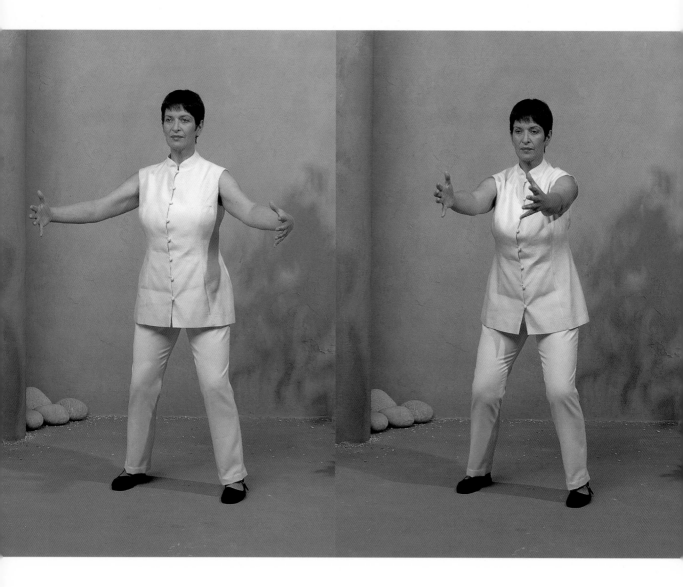

gathering up the sun

As its name suggests, this exercise involves visualizing and drawing in energy that feels warm and powerful like the sun. However, beginners should be cautious with this exercise until they have learnt how to feel the energy they are drawing in and how to ground it. Therefore, when drawing the energy up towards your chest, make sure you don't lift it higher than the chest area. The best way to avoid the energy travelling too high is to focus your attention on gathering energy in the lower *Dantian* (the point about 5 cm

(2 in) below the navel). Do the exercise slowly and keep your attention at *Dantian*. This will help you to feel grounded.

If you are disturbed during your Chi kung practice or are having trouble calming your thoughts, bring your focus to the *Dantian* point until you feel the warmth and energy there. It is important to remember that exercises such as this should not be done when you are feeling emotionally upset, have eaten too much, or do not have enough time to calm yourself and concentrate on the exercise.

Step 1

Adopting the basic Chi kung standing posture and with your palms facing forwards, bring your hands up to the centre of your body as though you are gathering up a ball of energy. I visualize myself lifting the rising sun up from the horizon.

Step 2

Stop when your hands are still a distance apart as if you were holding a ball, and feel the weight of the ball in your hands. Feel the weight evenly distributed through your legs and feet.

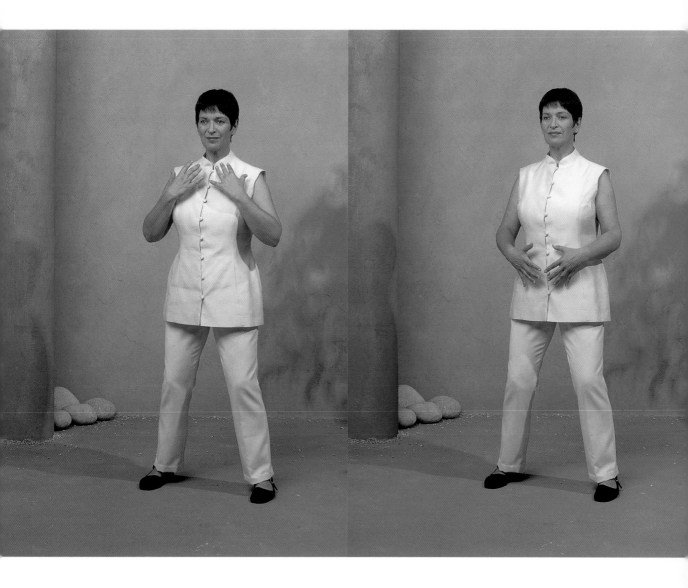

Now visualize yourself holding the warmth and energy of the sun between your hands.

Step 3
Breathing in, draw the energy ball towards your chest. When your hands are nearly touching your body turn your palms inwards to your body, fingertips pointing upwards.

Step 4
Now, breathing out, draw your hands down the front of your body. Imagine as you do this that you are covering yourself in warm, golden energy. Stop when your hands reach your navel, then hold and feel the energy at your centre. Feel the warmth in your hands and visualize all your organs having absorbed the golden energy. Move your hands outwards to the starting position at the side of your body, your palms facing your sides, and repeat the movement 4–6 times.

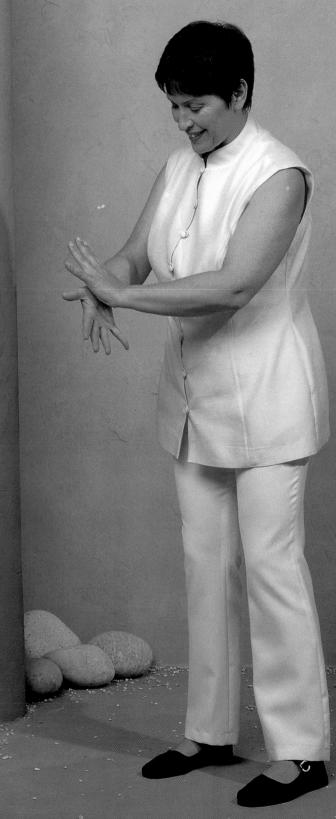

closing

Closing a Chi kung routine is very important. You should never just finish the exercises and continue with whatever you are doing without grounding the energy mentally and physically. Anyone who works with energy through other methods will vouch for the importance of finishing sessions properly and 'coming back into the world', so to speak. They will also tell you that there are a number of ways to do this. Although there are more exercises to come, this method of finishing your routine is placed here because the preceding five exercises form a core that benefit your general health, before beginning exercises for specific organs and conditions. However many exercises you do, always remember to include this closing sequence.

Step 1

If you have already done the preceding exercises, you should have noticed that your hands feel very warm, perhaps also tingly. This is *chi* energy that has gathered in your hands; it is important not to waste it.

Rub the palms of your hands together briskly. There is a point in the centre of each of your palms called *Laogong*. It is through these two points that we can transmit *chi* externally. In other healing practices such as Reiki, it is believed that these two points in the palms are minor *chakras*, through which the healing energy flows, and that there are two other minor chakras in the feet. This compares with the *Yongquan,* or kidney points, in Chi kung.

Now that you've rubbed your palms together and gathered the energy, rub them over your face as if washing yourself. This is excellent for your skin and makes you feel alert and wide awake. Run your fingers through your hair and hold your hands on your head to let some energy be absorbed there, too.

Step 2

Then, holding your hands out in front of you, let your wrists go limp. Shake your hands from the wrists, not the arms, as if you were shaking water off. You are getting rid of any harmful energy that is still there (see Releasing Stagnant *Chi*, Step 1, page 43).

Step 3

Now raise each foot in turn and shake it – this has the same effect as shaking your hands.

When you are doing this you could visualize the harmful *chi* either dissipating in the air or being buried in the ground. If you feel that you might fall over when you are doing this, hold on to something to steady yourself (see Releasing Stagnant *Chi*, Step 2, page 43).

Steps 4 a, b & c

Give a healing massage to all parts that need it – over the kidneys, small of the back, backs and sides of the knees, and over the hips; concentrate on where you have pain. Rub the major energy centres – the forehead, throat, back of the neck and both shoulders, centre of the chest, stomach, knees, ankles and sides of the feet. Slowly walk around for a while before resuming normal activities.

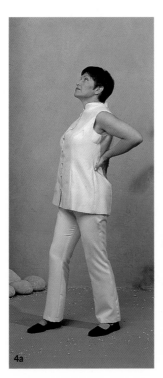
4a

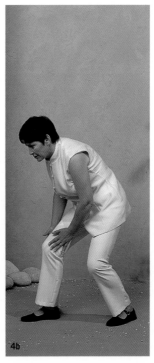
4b

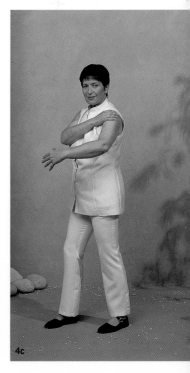
4c

connecting heaven and earth

This Chi kung exercise helps your spleen to work more efficiently. The spleen is an important element of our immune system. It helps to manufacture blood cells and destroy old ones as well as playing an integral part in iron metabolism. It also produces white blood cells and antibodies to fight infection.

The exercise is also good for preventing problems in the gastro-intestinal tract, as it promotes the flow of energy on both sides of the body, passing through the liver, gall bladder and stomach.

In addition, this is a particularly good exercise for women, since through menstruation and pregnancy they are more prone to anaemia, which is partly a result of an imbalance in the spleen's production and destruction of red blood cells, along with poor absorption of iron, which is also related to the spleen.

Remember when doing this and other exercises to ensure that your feet have good contact with the floor and that your knees are relaxed and slightly bent. You can help this by mentally visualizing your feet being sunken into the earth. This is important because a number of meridians either start or end in the feet, which is where we draw in our earth energy. You will also be more aware of contact with the earth if you wear, for example, Chinese slippers, which are worn for martial arts and allow you to feel more sensation in the feet than sports training shoes, which have thick soles.

Step 1

Relax your body and assume the Chi kung standing posture with your arms hanging in a natural position by your sides. Keep your breathing slow and steady. Now bring your hands together in front of your abdomen, with your palms facing up and the fingertips just touching, in a holding posture.

Step 2

Slowly raise your hands to chest height, as if you were holding a chalice or cup.

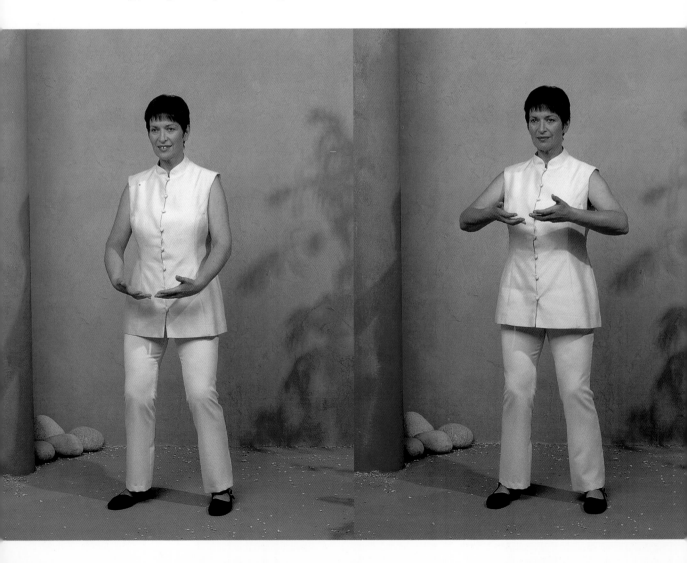

Step 3

Starting with your palms still held at chest height, bring your left arm above your head, and as you do this rotate your left palm to face upwards, as if you were holding up the sky, with your fingers pointing to the right-hand side of your body. Rotate your right palm to face the ground, bringing your right arm down to your side. Your hand should be at hip height, with your fingers pointing straight ahead and your palm pressing down.

Step 4

Bring your hands to abdomen level again and repeat the sequence, now with your right hand going above your head and your left by your side. When you are doing the exercise, you could visualize that the hand above your head is pushing the sky up, and the hand by your side is pushing a ball under water. Repeat the sequence for both sides 4–6 times.

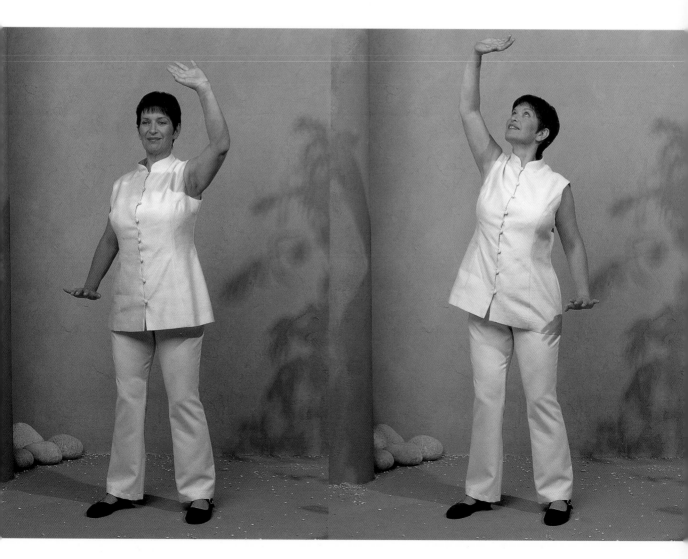

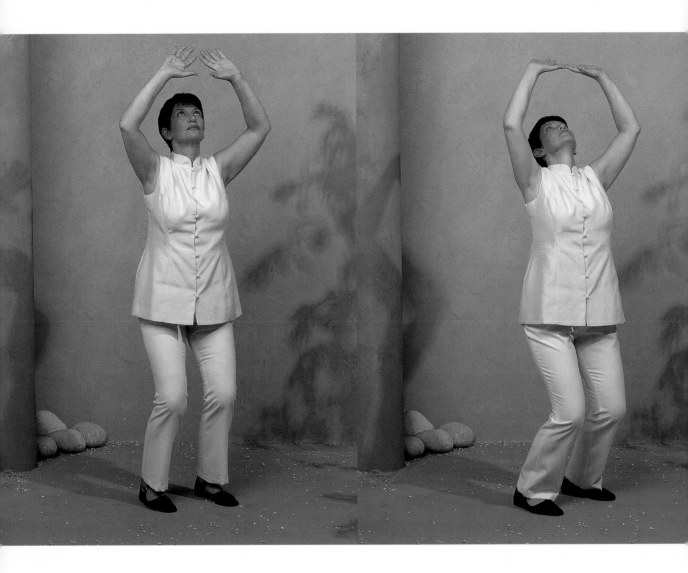

improving the liver

This exercise promotes the liver functions. The liver is the largest organ in our body, sitting on the right side just below the diaphragm which holds the lungs and heart in the upper part of the trunk. As part of the digestive system, its primary function is processing and extracting energy from the food we eat, and storing it as sugar, fat and protein. It also acts as a filter for toxins entering the body in any form. Like a filter in machinery, the liver must be working efficiently in order to remove toxins, otherwise they build up. The liver also secretes

bile, which is stored in the gall bladder. Problems with bile production often lead to gall-stones, especially for women, who suffer from this more frequently than men.

Your liver function will also benefit from removing unnecessary fat from your diet, which will then positively affect other body functions. If you want to accelerate the beneficial effects of Chi kung on your body, the best way to do it is not through making yourself practise more and more Chi kung, but through combining Chi kung with an improved diet. Personally, I have

found that practising Chi kung daily has made me more aware of what I am eating because I am more aware of my body. I also find myself desiring healthier foods that would not have been my first choice before I started practising Chi kung. This is a good example of the way in which Chi kung can change your consciousness without involving the will.

Step 1

Before starting, assume the standing posture (see page 47), with your arms relaxed by your sides. Then bring your hands

together at abdomen level in a holding position, palms facing upwards. Slowly raise your hands to chest height as if gathering up a bowl. When your hands reach your chest, slowly rotate your palms over to face the earth and, as you do so, bring your fingertips loosely together. Holding your hands in that shape, bring your arms up above your head, with your palms facing the sky.

Step 2

Tilt your head backwards, look up through the heart shape that your hands have formed and

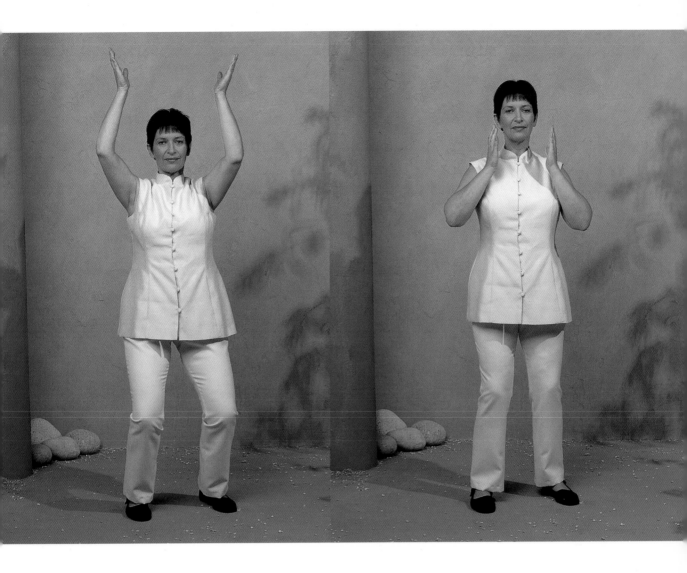

gather the heaven energy in
your hands.

Step 3
When you sense that you have
gathered enough energy into
your hands, bring your head
back into the normal position
and look straight ahead.

At the same time, make your
hands into a funnel shape just
above your head, and have the
palms facing each other but at
an angle.

Step 4
With your mind, lead the column
of energy you have gathered in

your hands down through the
crown of your head and through
the body to the navel or *Dantian*,
and keep it there. At the same
time bring your hands down to
the holding position by following
the shape of your body. Repeat
4–6 times.

relax & visualize

As you will have gathered, being in a relaxed state is an important element of successfully practising Chi kung. When you are tense, your mind is unable to focus on what you are doing and you tend to go through the exercises without really experiencing them. It is undoubtedly very difficult to clear all the endless chatter that goes on in our minds even when we are not feeling particularly stressed, as anyone who has tried 'clearing the mind' for meditation will probably agree. We are so used to multi-tasking in our minds that we find it impossible to think of only one thing at a time. Basically we have to retrain our minds to do this and there are a few basic techniques, all of which have numerous stylistic variations.

Some people focus on the breath at the point where it enters and leaves the nose. Others focus on an object – a

candle flame, for example. Another method is the use of a mantra, as in Transcendental Meditation. They are all different ways of achieving this one aim – getting the mind to relax and to focus.

In Chi kung, the mind leads *chi* energy, which is why visualization is such an important part of the exercises. Those that follow are based on breathing and on visualization because these techniques are central to Chi kung. Two are static and one is a meditation that uses movement. They can be used before starting your warm-ups and exercise routine, or you may prefer, as I do, to perform them at the end of your practice session. You can also use them independently of Chi kung – the breathing meditation is very useful if you can't get to sleep, for example.

meditating on breath

This short meditation will also help you to develop the ability to open your Third Eye, another name for the sixth *chakra* and centre of psychic perception.

Lie down or sit with your spine well supported and relaxed. Begin by letting all the tension out of your body. To do this, work from the top of your head to your feet down your front, letting go of tension in all your muscles. Repeat down your back and then your sides.

Now focus on your breath, counting each out-breath from one to four. When you get to your fourth out-breath, begin at one again. Don't try to control your breathing – as you become more relaxed the breaths will naturally become longer. Focus on counting instead. If you are very relaxed you will soon enter a deep meditative state and may even fall asleep.

moving meditation

Stand up to do this exercise and, ideally, play some quiet, rhythmic music.

Imagine yourself to be a reed standing in water or a plant growing at the bottom of the ocean. Feel yourself being moved by the flowing current of water around you, bending you but supporting you, pushing you from side to side as you sway. Now feel yourself naturally attracted to the light above the water and feel yourself growing up from your roots towards it. At the same time enjoy the feeling of being anchored to the earth or sea-bed by your roots. Feel yourself stretching and swaying simultaneously to the music, and let your mind float without focusing on any other images. When you are ready, open your eyes, rub your face and shake your hands to return you to the room.

visualization

You can either learn this exercise by reading it several times, or by making a tape for yourself.

Lie or sit in a relaxed position and let the tension out of your body. See yourself getting into a boat and floating down a river. Look out for a tree where you can moor your boat, and when you have tied up the boat, stay in it for a little while and listen to the water lapping at the sides.

When you are ready, climb out of the boat and walk up the riverbank into a field. You walk across the field and through a forest until you find a house in a clearing. This is your house and it can be a hut or a mansion. Go inside it. When you do, make a note of what the house is like inside. How is it decorated? Does it seem big or small inside?

Enter one of the rooms. Someone will come to meet you there. Who is it? A friend, a

parent or a stranger? Ask them a question and they will give you an answer, or perhaps they will simply give you a gift.

Now say goodbye to them and return to your boat, walking back through the forest and across the field. Note any changes on your return journey. Is the light or weather different? Has the forest or field changed? Get back into your boat and float back to where you started, and when you are ready, open your eyes and stretch all your muscles to relax them as you come back into the present time.

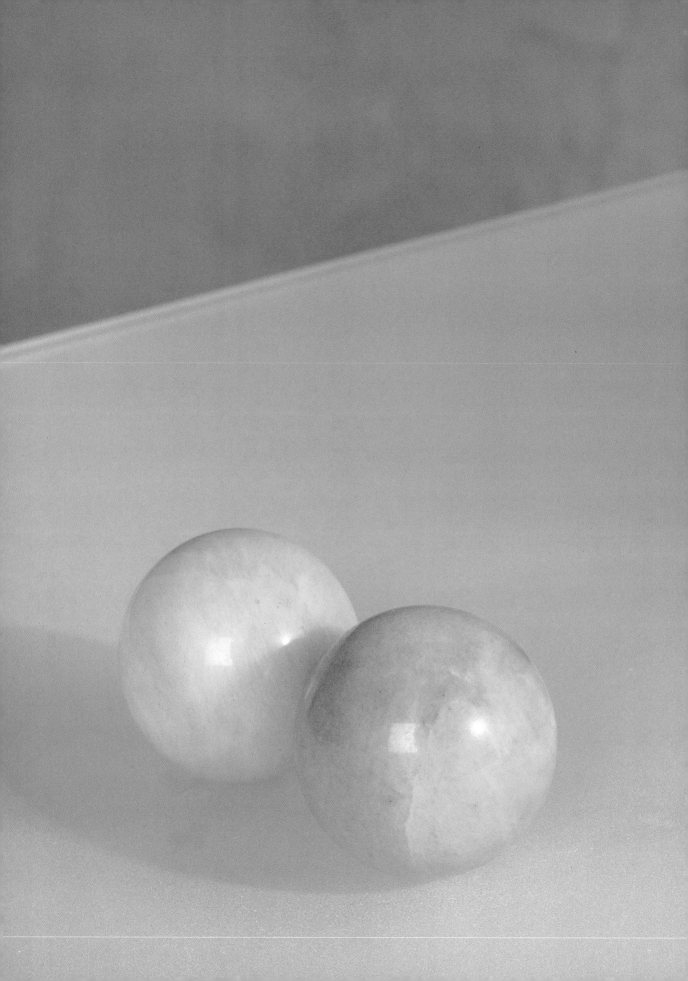

chi kung &
sexual health

In Chi kung, sexual health or good sexual energy is not simply associated
with improving or increasing a person's sexual desire or performance. It is
recognized that sexual energy is interdependent with the energy in the whole
of the body and that it is not something that operates in isolation. In the West,
by contrast, we tend not to connect our sexual energy with our general health.
We also believe that sexual energy is only for use in our sex lives, whereas in
Chi kung, sexual energy can be cultivated and directed to improve physical
and mental health. In the West we also have no concept of losing or wasting
sexual energy, whereas in the East, conserving sexual energy – but not through
abstinence from sex – is an important part of promoting longevity.

sexual energy to improve your health

As we grow older, we become less able to acquire the energy our bodies need. In youth we get all we require from external sources, such as air and food, and through exercise. At the same time we expend only three-quarters of it daily, which is why children in particular often just don't know what to do with all that extra energy.

When we get older, we still need the same amount of energy each day to enable us to function, but we are no longer so good at acquiring it from external sources. The result is an energy deficit, and to compensate we start to use energy from our internal organs. If we keep drawing energy from these internal reserves without replenishing it, we cause our organs to age and atrophy at a faster rate. To stop this we need to learn both how to draw in more energy and to conserve and cultivate that energy once we have acquired it. Practising Chi kung is one way to do this.

The energy with which we are born is called *jing*, which is generative or creative energy. This is your innate energy that is essential for all your physical functions. *Jing* resides in the lower body, but is stored in all the body tissues, particularly in the kidneys, and also in the sperm and ova (eggs). The other energies in the body – the *chi* and *shen* – are dependent on it. That is why many Chi kung exercises focus on storing and cultivating energy in the lower *Dantian* area, just below the navel, because it is important to build up your *jing* first. It will also help you to remember that your kidneys are the source of sexuality, virility and fertility, and all sexual disorders are connected to the kidney system. Nourishing your kidneys is therefore important for your sex life as well as for your general health.

The Taoists believed that there are two main ways in which men and women lose energy. For men it is through ejaculation during sexual intercourse, and for women it is through menstruation. In his book *Cultivating Female Sexual Energy*, Mantak Chia states that during her life only two of a woman's eggs on average are used to create children, while the rest are eliminated. These eggs contain sexual energy and their elimination through menstruation results in the loss of between 30 and 40 per cent of her principal energy. Similarly, every time a man ejaculates, he is losing the energy contained in his sperm.

The Taoists also believed that sexual energy is the only type of energy that can be significantly increased. Therefore, if we want to replenish the *jing* energy that fuels our biological functions, we should conserve and recycle sexual energy to do that. The method of doing this is through exercises that allow us to turn orgasmic energy inward instead of outward, as is normally the case.

In Chi kung there are two approaches to developing sexual energy – sole cultivation and dual cultivation. As you might expect, sole cultivation means working alone while dual cultivation means working with your partner. Using the sole cultivation route removes the necessity of being in a sexual relationship in order to work with your sexual energy, and even those in a relationship are advised to work alone initially in order to perfect the different techniques for men and women. Also, if you want to practise sexual Chi kung but your partner doesn't, you can still do it on your own.

sole and dual cultivation

During sexual intercourse couples exchange energy. Through this energy exchange each person is 'balanced' by the other, and that is an integral element of sexual desire, albeit a largely unconscious one. In dual cultivation using sexual Chi kung, the couple learn exercises that control this exchange of yin and yang energy, and through practice eventually experience the exchange of *chi* at the soul or spirit level.

The aim of sole cultivation is to preserve sexual energy and learn how to draw it up the Governor channel (which runs up from the base of the spine, over the head and finishes on the upper lip) to higher centres. By practising the exercises alone you will become more attuned to your own responses and therefore able to control your own energy better, so that when you work with a partner, you are familiar with what is happening to you. For a woman, the exercises teach her how to strengthen the sexual organs and tissues and how to use breathing techniques to draw orgasmic energy up into the other organs. For men, the main aim of sexual Chi kung is to control the ejaculation of semen while still achieving orgasm. The exercises that follow will give you a taste of this fascinating aspect of Chi kung.

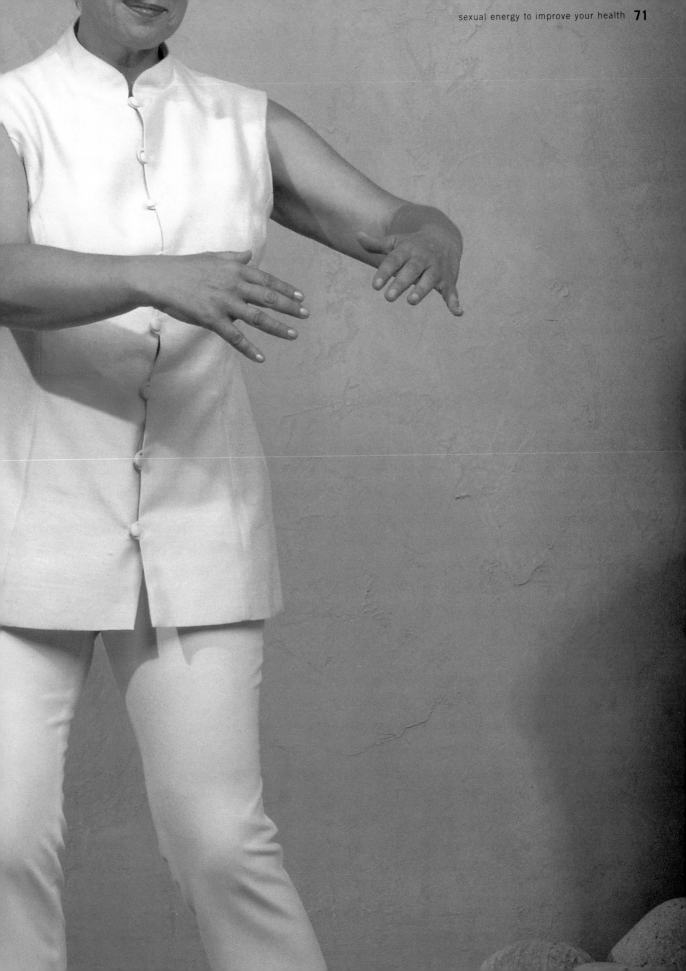

replenishing the kidneys

According to Chinese medical thinking, the kidneys play a vital part in determining men's virility and women's fertility. Strengthening the kidneys will also improve your general health and this in turn will enhance your sexual feelings and desire as well as the pleasure you derive. The basic exercise is for everyone and it can be included in your daily set of exercises. It will help you to remove toxins from the kidney and bladder system and tone up the muscles in the back of your legs as well as increasing your sexual pleasure. The exercise can also, it is reputed, help prevent hair loss in men.

Step 1
Stand in the Chi kung posture, relaxed and breathing naturally. Begin by focusing your attention on the kidney points (*Yongquan*) in the soles of your feet which connect you to the earth energy.

Step 2
Then, with your knees straight, bend over to touch your toes with your fingers, breathing out as you bend.

Step 3
Hold on to your big toe (even if you are wearing shoes). Some people will be unable to do this, and you should not try to force yourself to touch your toes, for the aim is always to feel relaxed. Instead, bend your knees as you reach down with your hands as far as is comfortable for both your back and your legs – you will still benefit from the posture. While in this position, visualize *chi* energy flowing up your spine from your perineum (*Huiyin* point) to the crown of your head (*Baihui* point). Hold the energy there for 2–3 seconds and then visualize the energy travelling down to the centre of your palms (*Laogong* points). Now breathe in and slowly raise your body until you are completely upright again. As you are doing this visualize your hands filled with energy.

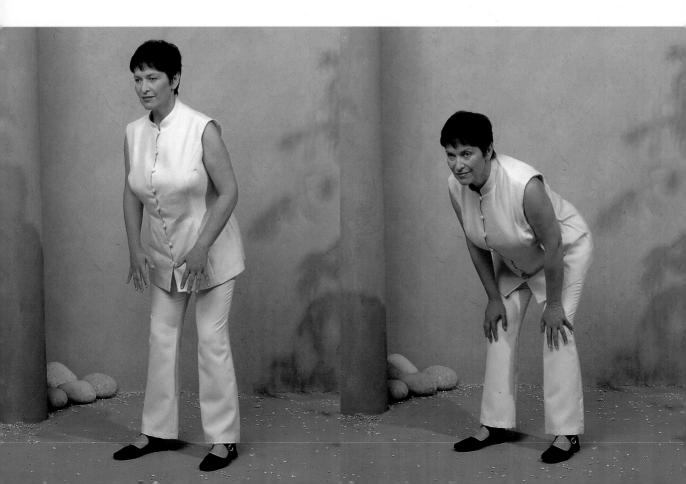

Step 4

Now place both your palms on your kidneys and arch your back slightly so that your kidneys can absorb the energy from your hands. First visualize the energy entering your kidneys and nourishing them. Then visualize the energy travelling to your bladder and sex organs to revitalize them. When you have done this, adopt your original posture, with your arms by your side. Repeat the exercise 6 times.

Step 5 (optional)

The kidneys tend to get clogged up with sediment if they are not efficiently filtering out waste material from the blood and this can result in kidney stones. To loosen up this sediment and enhance the exercise above, you can do the following. Form your hands into loose fists as in the exercise Knocking at the Door of Life (see page 42), then hit your kidneys with the back of your fists, using the arm-swinging action – but only hit them as hard as is comfortable for you.

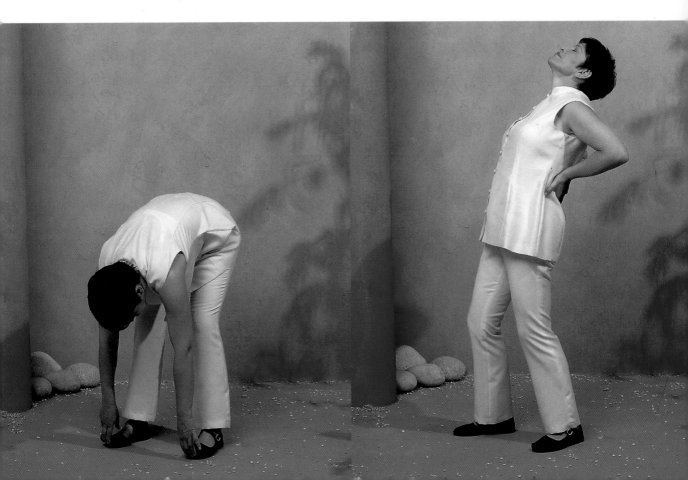

preparation

If you are going to set aside time
to work with your sexual energy
as separate from other Chi kung
exercises, you will probably find
it helpful to spend a little time
before you do the exercises,
focusing on building your energy
in the lower *Dantian*. To do this,
lie down for 5–10 minutes, or
longer if you wish, and visualize
each in-breath coming to that
point. Remember to breathe into
your abdomen so that it rises
and falls, not your chest. Keep
your breathing relaxed and do
not try to take too much air in.
You will soon feel the area
become warm and energized.
Now you are ready to circulate
the accumulated energy.

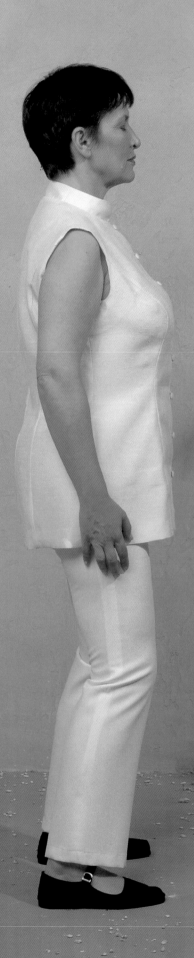

circulating sexual energy

In ancient cultures, particularly those of Egypt, India and China, women were taught techniques for circulating sexual energy around their bodies. Using these techniques encourages women to make use of their sexual energy for themselves first and in relationships second. The exercises also offer women a way of redefining their sexual selves by moving the focus of sexual pleasure away from the genital orgasm to a whole-body experience.

The exercises described here are for beginners. People interested in developing expertise in either sole or dual cultivation of sexual energy should consult other books dedicated to the subject. The author Mantak Chia's works are particularly recommended for techniques such as Ovarian Breathing for women and techniques for preventing ejaculation in men, which is seen as their main means of energy loss.

the microcosmic orbit

This is a simplified form of an advanced Chi kung exercise. It will probably take some practice before you actually feel the energy moving through this entire circuit. Don't concern yourself if you don't feel it initially – just mentally take the energy around and the sensation will follow. If you find that too much energy is becoming stuck in your head after doing this exercise, resulting in dizziness or a headache, take the energy down to your feet and allow it to flow into the earth.

Step 1
Assume the sitting posture or, if you prefer, stand. Keeping your eyes completely or partially closed will help your concentration. Keep your tongue pressed against your hard palate.

Step 2
First take the energy from the point just below your navel to your perineum, between the vagina and the anus, and contract the muscles there.

Step 3
Now take the energy from the perineum to the base of your spine, and from there guide the energy up your spine, past the back of the heart to the neck and up the back of your head to your crown. Visualize the energy starting to flow down from the crown to the tongue which, placed against the roof of your mouth, connects two circuits. Now the energy flows down the central route in the front of your body back to the perineum.

breathing in pleasure

It is thought that one of the main obstacles to a woman achieving orgasm with a partner is fear – fear of losing self-control. But fear is only a learned response and that response can be reprogrammed, and one method of doing it is through breathing. As discussed earlier, one of the responses to stress is increased shallow breathing and slow, calm breathing is needed to reverse that response. The abdominal Breathing Technique (see pages 48–49) can be used during masturbation to increase the feelings of pleasure. Remember that every time you breathe out you are breathing out fear, and as you breathe in become more aware of the pleasurable sensations in your body. As you feel yourself approach orgasm, use your breath to take you into it, breathing past any emotional blocks that are holding you back. In this way you move out of your head and into your body, which is the key part of the problem for most people.

the triangle

This exercise, which improves the urinary and reproductive systems generally, can be done by both men and women. It has been found to be effective for premature ejaculation and impotence in men and for infertility problems and irregular or painful periods for women. The exercise involves circulating energy around the abdomen.

Begin in either the standing or sitting posture. As you inhale, pull up the walls of the anus by squeezing the muscles together. Now imagine that you can feel the flow of energy from the *Huiyin* point, which is just in front of the anus. The energy flows from this point through the anus and up the spine to your *Mingmen* point, which is at the centre of the waist, between your kidneys.

Now, instead of taking the energy on up the spine, as in the Microcosmic Orbit (see page 75), visualize the energy travelling straight from the *Mingmen* point through the body to *Dantian*, the energy point around your navel. Exhaling, direct the energy from *Dantian* down to *Huiyin* again, pause, breathe in, and direct the energy round the triangular circuit again. The area between these three points, *Huiyin*, *Mingmen* and *Dantian*, will warm up after several repetitions of the circuit.

Begin by repeating the circuit 4–6 times, building up to 12, 24 or 36 in time.

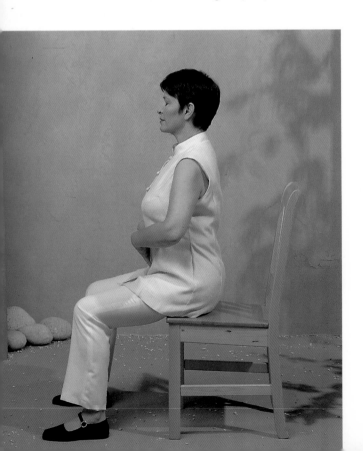

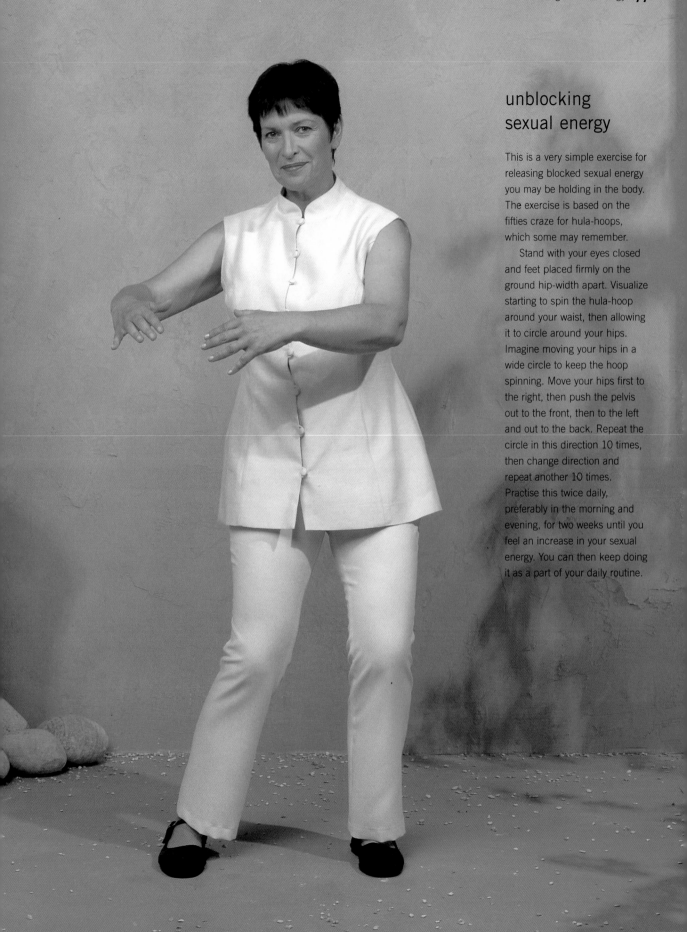

unblocking sexual energy

This is a very simple exercise for releasing blocked sexual energy you may be holding in the body. The exercise is based on the fifties craze for hula-hoops, which some may remember.

Stand with your eyes closed and feet placed firmly on the ground hip-width apart. Visualize starting to spin the hula-hoop around your waist, then allowing it to circle around your hips. Imagine moving your hips in a wide circle to keep the hoop spinning. Move your hips first to the right, then push the pelvis out to the front, then to the left and out to the back. Repeat the circle in this direction 10 times, then change direction and repeat another 10 times. Practise this twice daily, preferably in the morning and evening, for two weeks until you feel an increase in your sexual energy. You can then keep doing it as a part of your daily routine.

chi kung for women

All people are governed by natural cycles – women more obviously than men. Every 28 days, as the moon passes through its phases, the *chi* in the human body also completes a cycle up the back and down the front of the body in the Governor and Conception channels. When the moon is full the *chi* is at the crown of the head, and when the moon is dark, the *chi* is at the perineum. This echoes a woman's menstrual cycle.

When the *chi* is blocked or insufficiently strong, imbalance occurs, resulting in menstrual, menopausal and hormonal problems. The physical and emotional symptoms of these are experienced by more women than is necessary. Chi kung offers women a way to strengthen the flow of *chi* and restore harmony to their bodies naturally.

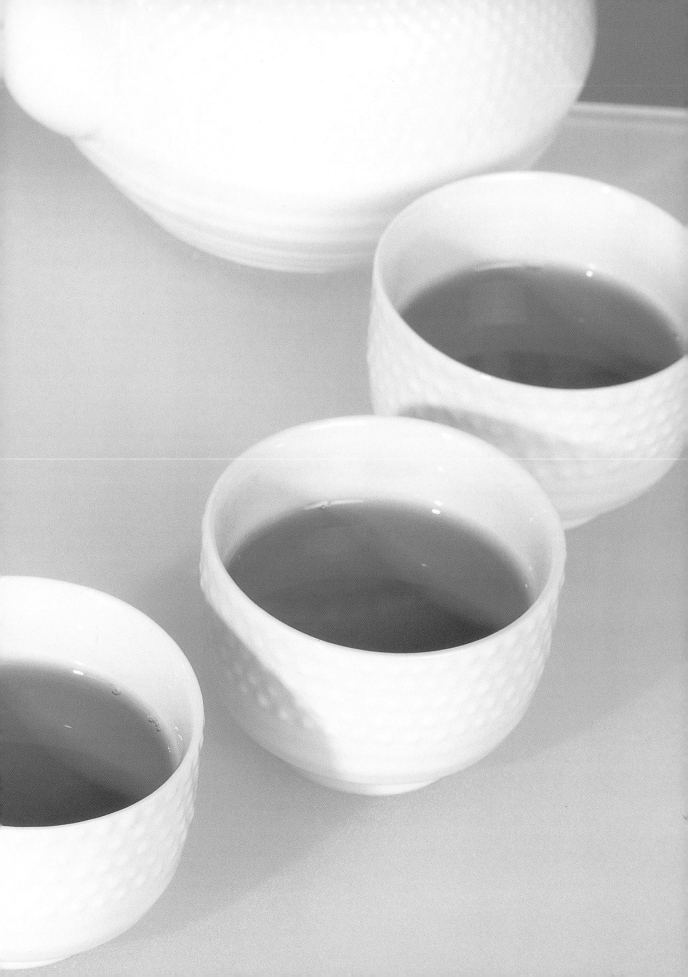

natural help for women

A woman's life has well-defined stages, which may be described as daughter, mother, grandmother – or, metaphorically, as princess, queen and empress. With each transition a woman increases her personal power, until post-menopause she is at the pinnacle of self-knowing – the empress and wise woman of her world. However, this isn't quite the story that most women have been told, though happily it is one that is rapidly gaining a following among women as they reclaim their inner strength and innate femininity, a femininity that is not one defined by male culture. This is a reversal of the values of contemporary Western culture, which place youthful energy and beauty over and above the spiritual energy and wisdom that can only be acquired over time. Using Chi kung, women can cultivate their energy on all levels, so that at each stage in their lives and with every change they can live their lives fully.

menstruation and pms

The move from girlhood into womanhood is defined by the beginning of menstruation, and for the next 40 or so years the woman's life is a series of monthly cycles, recorded in diaries or as dates circled on calendars. For some this transition is a positive event to be celebrated, but for all too many it is something frightening, something to be hidden and something to be endured. Perhaps this is because in the West we have no ceremony to celebrate the passage from girlhood to womanhood, and because girls and young women are often given to believe that menstruation is a negative interruption in their lives for several days every month. As they start menstruating, girls are given these messages which make them anticipate problems, and perhaps that is why so many of them do go on to experience painful menstruation. Also, before the onset of each period, there are the mood swings, tiredness, headaches, outbreaks of acne, cravings for chocolate and the host of other symptoms that are now given the umbrella term Pre-menstrual Syndrome, or PMS for short. The symptoms normally occur in the second half of the cycle, between ovulation and menstruation, and it is estimated that about 80 per cent of women experience at least one symptom every month, although individual experience varies widely.

What causes PMS? In simplified terms, orthodox medicine says it is caused by hormone imbalance, and Chinese medicine says it is an imbalance of the spleen, kidneys and liver. Other medical systems have their own way of defining it, but whichever medical approach you choose the key concept that underlies each definition is that of imbalance. When the menstrual cycle is in natural harmony, women will experience the different stages of the cycle but not in an unpleasant way as is the case with PMS. Instead they will be aware of the changes in physical and mental energy. In the days between menstruation and ovulation, a woman's energy is rising and outgoing, making it a time to start new projects and to do things out in the world. The time between ovulation and menstruation is a time of increasingly moving inward in both thoughts and actions, a slowing-down so that by the time menstruation arrives the woman is ready to retreat inside herself for a few days, resting and reflecting before the next phase. If women observe this pattern they can organize their lives to maximize the energy available to them.

Chi kung helps women to find the internal physiological balance that removes the symptoms of PMS and, at the same time, makes them more aware of the nature of the creative energy they have and how best they can use it. It teaches a woman to value quietness, and to respect it, when that is what she needs. It also teaches her awareness of creative strengths, how to share them and the best time to use them. In other words, it helps her express herself as a woman in every way.

the menopause

Then there is the menopause. This is something that is feared even more than menstruation, since in Western culture it is portrayed as an almost life-ending event. In the last two decades, orthodox medicine has found a way of preventing menopausal symptoms through Hormone Replacement Therapy (HRT). In the absence of widespread and affordable access to more natural ways of controlling menopausal symptoms, and in a society that openly denigrates the symptoms by making them a source of jokes, it is not surprising that many women turn to HRT. But in Chi kung and in Chinese medical philosophy, the menopause is seen as the time when *jing*, or biological energy, transforms into spirit, and with it comes spiritual wisdom. Therefore, menopause is something to be welcomed, not avoided. The uncomfortable symptoms, however, are unwelcome and can be alleviated using Chi kung and, if necessary, herbal prescriptions that act in a similar way to HRT.

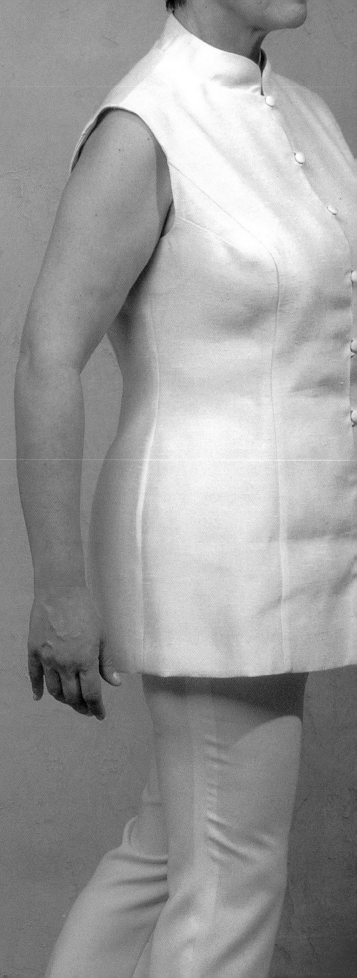

when women should avoid chi kung

There are times when women should be cautious about practising Chi kung, although they do not need to stop completely. These times are during menstruation and pregnancy. In the case of menstruation, some women find that their periods become heavier after some months of practice or that practising Chi kung during menstruation increases the flow. In both cases all that is required is to keep the energy around or slightly above the navel area in exercises where you are asked to push the energy down towards the earth. Instead, as you practise, keep your attention focused on the heart and lungs, circulating the energy down the arms to the hands.

In the case of pregnancy more caution is required and you should especially avoid pushing the energy down below the lower *Dantian*. Do not practise the more strenuous exercises or ones that require you to lower your body very far. It is also advised that you do not practise abdominal breathing (see page 48), but that you revert to your natural method of breathing while practising.

If you are in any doubt about which exercises to practise, while pregnant it is best to consult a Chi kung teacher, who will be able to advise you as to which are suitable.

menopause & hormone regulation

Between 25 and 50 per cent of all women do not suffer from menopausal symptoms at all, and those who do may suffer from one or two only. These include hot flushes, decreased libido, insomnia, irritability, depression and osteoporosis.

The lead-up period to the menopause lasts approximately 10–15 years and the average age when the menopause itself occurs is 51 years. During this time the ovaries gradually produce less and less oestrogen. It is the lack of oestrogen that causes most of the physical and emotional symptoms, and it is also this lack that leaves post-menopausal women more vulnerable to heart disease and osteoporosis. Hormone Replacement Therapy (HRT) can be used to supplement the lack of both oestrogen and progesterone, although women who have had their uterus removed can be treated with oestrogen only. There are of course side effects associated with HRT, but for many the benefits – protection against heart disease, improved sexual functioning and the preservation of more youthful looks – outweigh any disadvantages.

Chi kung exercises can help mitigate the effects of slowly declining oestrogen levels and help regulate menstruation in the years before the menopause. A study at the Shanghai Chi kung Institute tested blood oestrogen levels in men and women after a two-month course in Chi kung and compared them with a control group not doing Chi kung. The control group showed no changes in hormone levels, but in the Chi kung group levels of oestrogen in the men dropped, while in the women it rose, particularly in those over 45 years.

Chi kung may also delay the onset of menopause, and female Chi kung masters have been known to conceive in their sixties, although Chinese medical philosophy does not advocate motherhood in the forties or after, in the belief that children born of older parents have a weaker constitution.

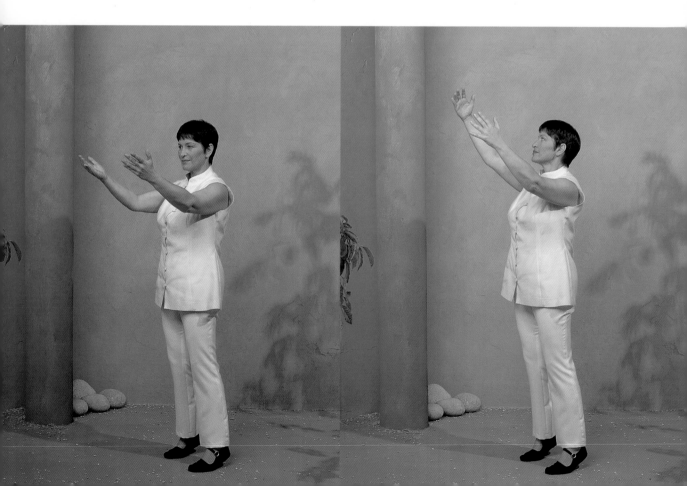

regulating hormone levels

This exercise is effective in both helping with hormone regulation and for preventing osteoporosis, which is a result of low levels of oestrogen. It will be most effective when practised along with the warm-ups and eight-exercise Chi kung routine (see pages 38–45 and 50–68). You can extend this exercise into a walking routine like the one which follows and include the Shower of Light described in the daily routine (see page 52).

Step 1

Begin by taking up the standing position, looking straight ahead and having your arms relaxed by your sides.

Slowly raise your hands to bring them above your head, your palms facing the sky. As you bring your hands up, rise up on to the balls of your feet.

Step 2

Continue raising your hands and stretching upwards.

Step 3

Once your hands are right up above your head, turn your palms around so that when you come to lower them they will be facing the earth.

Step 4

Swing your hands back down to your sides as you bounce down on to your heels. Allow the downward movement of your arms to complete its full, natural swing.

Keep your arms relaxed and slightly rounded as you do the exercise, never rigid and straight. Repeat 4–6 times to begin with, before building up to 12, 24 or 36 times. As you become more familiar with the exercise you can also build up a faster rhythm. It might help you if you practise while listening to some music with a suitably paced beat.

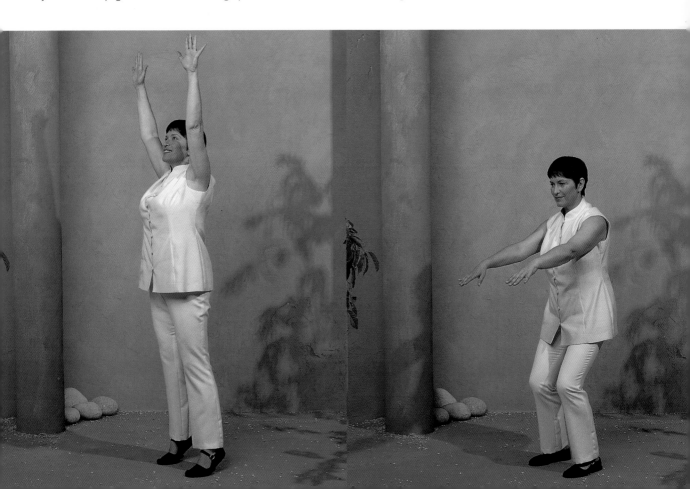

osteoporosis

After the age of 35 the body creates less new bone and also becomes less efficient at storing calcium. Osteoporosis can affect men but it is primarily associated with women, because women have about 30 per cent less bone mass than men to begin with. With osteoporosis, the bones lose their density, becoming fragile and brittle. Unfortunately, there are no symptoms until the disease is well advanced, when even a coughing fit can cause a fracture in the ribs.

Fractures of the wrist, spine and hips are the most common problems associated with osteoporosis. A fractured wrist is the easiest to tolerate. A fracture in the spine will inflict severe pain for several weeks and will cause the spine to contract, resulting in loss of height. Fractures to the hip are most serious and may even cause death. One of the reasons for this is not the osteoporosis itself but the fact that an elderly person may have to lie on the floor for a long time waiting for help to arrive, whilst suffering from shock. Treatment and recovery rates have improved in recent years, but still a significant number of people die within six months of a bone fracture, while the independence of those that live is severely reduced.

Apart from the loss of oestrogen with age, other personal factors are thought to be predictors of osteoporosis. Late onset of menstruation is one, as is early menopause, that is, before the age of 45. Smoking, low weight to height ratio as well as having had either anorexia or an over-active thyroid gland are also likely contributors to the problem, as well as long-term treatment with corticosteroids. Those women least likely to suffer from osteoporosis will be slightly overweight and will have had more sex hormones than average circulating in their bodies. This means that they will have started menstruating earlier than average and reached menopause much later than average. In between they will have had several children and breast-fed them all. They will not have smoked and will not have had a seriously debilitating disease such as asthma or arthritis. They will probably also have used the contraceptive pill.

However, even if you do not fit that description there are still many ways of preventing osteoporosis. The Chi kung exercises that help to prevent it are, like many of the exercises recommended by physiotherapists, based on weight-bearing. One of the best prevention methods for osteoporosis is vigorous walking. The 'walking Chi kung' exercise (right) is rather more gentle and is therefore suitable for both prevention and to aid those who have already been diagnosed. The bouncing exercise in the warm-up routine (see page 38) is also beneficial for osteoporosis, as is the exercise preceding this. The exercise focusing on the kidneys (see pages 74–75) will also help, and clicking your teeth together several times a day will help both bones and teeth.

clicking teeth

Relax your lips and click your teeth together lightly 36 times. This will create a lot of saliva in your mouth, which you should try to swallow in three gulps. This strengthens both the teeth and gums and when the teeth get stronger the bones also get stronger.

walking chi kung

You will need space to do this, but an average-sized room with furniture should suffice. Having done your warm-ups and other exercises, including meditation, you might do this at the end of your routine.

Step 1
Start in a relaxed standing position. Ensure that you are aware of your *Baihui* point and that your head feels stretched up to the sky from that point. Now

start to walk, keeping the eyes focused ahead and not looking down at your feet. Walk with a deliberate, slightly rolling motion. Start by moving your left foot forward and firmly placing your heel on the ground. It is important to make the connection firm as your heel connects with your sexual energy.

Step 2
Now move forward by pushing your weight down on to the front

of your right foot, making sure the kidney point is firmly connected to the floor. The kidney points are called the Bubbling Spring (*Yongquan*), and the rolling movement while you are walking comes with the feeling of springing upward off these points.

Step 3
Repeat the process with your left foot, and focus on the kidney points as you walk.

Step 4
If you are walking indoors, walk in a circle with slow, deliberate steps, letting your *Baihui* point on the crown lead you.

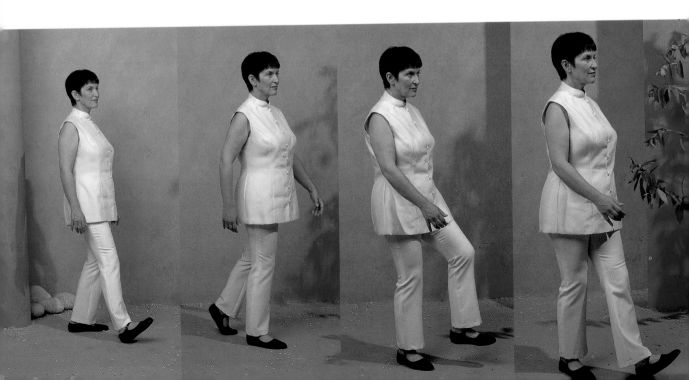

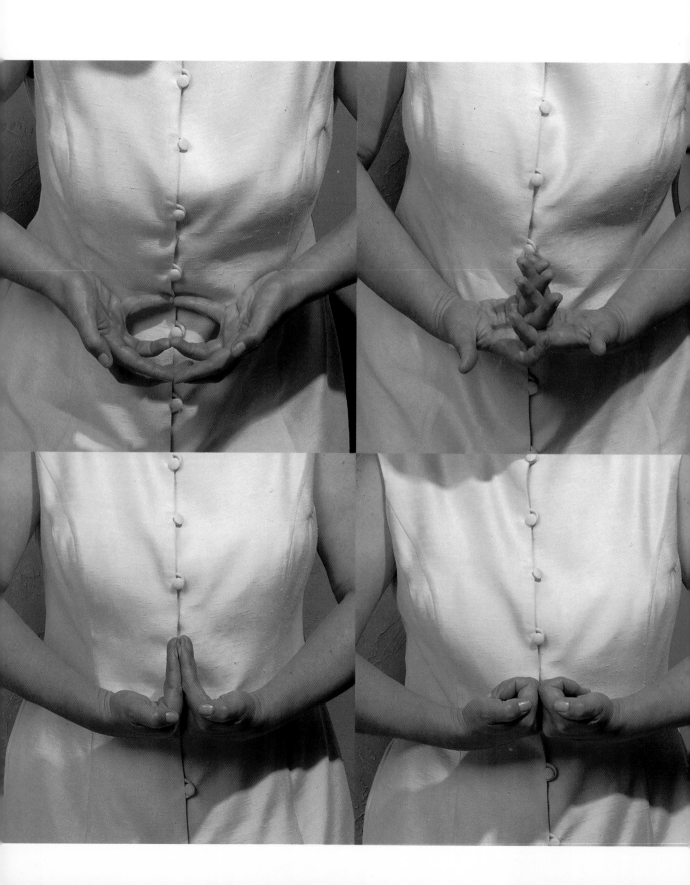

incontinence

One of the symptoms of the hormonal changes associated with the menopause is incontinence. This is due to the drying and thinning of the vaginal wall, which in turn can weaken the entrance to the bladder. Sudden and embarrassing leakage of urine can be caused by laughter, coughing or sneezing. This can also happen after childbirth and the same technique is used to prevent and cure both of these problems as well as preventing prolapse of the uterus, another menopausal symptom.

The Basic Pelvic-floor Exercise below is widely used in ante- and post-natal classes. It has also traditionally been used to enhance sexual pleasure, as it maintains strength in the vaginal muscles. One of the great advantages of this exercise is that you can practise it as often as you like every day without anyone knowing that you are doing it, though the best way to practise it and test it out is by trying to stop urinating in mid-flow by contracting your muscles as described here.

In addition to the simple and traditional pelvic-floor exercise, the other version below includes visualization and awareness of energy.

basic pelvic-floor exercise

Sitting or standing are the best positions for this exercise, but it can also be done lying down. Rhythmically contract and release the pelvic-floor muscles. When you contract the muscles, hold them for a few seconds and squeeze as if you were stopping the flow of urine. Repeat this as many times a day as you can. When you become proficient at this exercise you will be able to contract different parts of the muscles in that area separately so that you can control different parts of the vagina.

the lift

So-called because it helps to visualize a lift or elevator going up while doing the exercise, this has the same basic actions as the Basic Pelvic-floor Exercise.

Sitting or standing, start to contract the pelvic-floor muscles but imagine you are pulling the muscles only up to the first floor and hold them there. Now pull the muscles in a little more, go up another floor and hold. Keep contracting and holding them in stages until the muscles are squeezed tight. As you do this visualize your energy flowing down to the kidney points in your feet, then up to your coccyx at the base of the spine, from there to the *Mingmen* between the kidneys and then to

the urethra, the canal through which urine passes from the bladder out of the body.

If your pelvic floor is weak it may help to tighten the muscles around the anus and feel you are pulling the pelvic floor up that way. Then visualize shutting the lift door and going up. Hold the lift at the first floor and imagine letting more people in, then go to the second floor. As you get stronger you may be able to go up to the third floor. As you release the muscles, imagine the lift is descending, stopping at each floor to let people out. While doing either version, keep your body weight on the soles of your feet to increase the connection with the earth.

skin rejuvenation

One of the great benefits of Chi kung is that it improves the look and feel of your skin after even a relatively short period of regular practice. There are two reasons for this. One is that Chi kung improves the flow of *chi* energy in all parts of the body, and this of course is reflected in the appearance of skin, hair and eyes. The second reason for the improvement in the tone and suppleness of the skin is the use of abdominal breathing during Chi kung exercises. The lungs and skin are our connection with the external world and both absorb *chi* from it. The lungs breathe in air and absorb the *chi* in it, while the skin absorbs energy from the light of the sun, moon and stars. The lungs breathe old, stale energy out and the skin discharges toxins in the form of sweat. The relationship between the lungs and the skin is such that healthy breathing means healthy skin. In Chinese medicine, the lungs, skin and large intestine are associated with the element of metal and with sorrow and grief.

When practising Chi kung, the benefits you gain progress through five levels: skin, flesh, meridians, bones and internal organs. Therefore, you will see the benefits in your skin first as the improved flow of energy promotes better blood circulation. This allows toxins to be more easily eliminated through the skin and results in renewed vitality in the skin tissue. Apart from enjoying this improvement for its own sake, it is also visible proof that Chi kung is working and encourages you to continue. If you have long-term skin problems they will take a little longer to clear, but be patient and you will see improvements in these, too.

Self-massage is an important part of Chi kung, the Meridian Massage (see page 44) being one form of it. The facial massage outlined here utilizes acupoints on the face and will not only improve the appearance your skin but will also benefit other organs in the body.

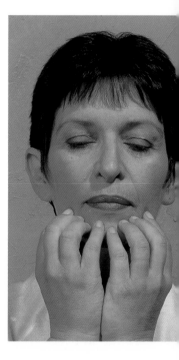

facial massage

Step 1
Hook your thumbs under your chin and massage your chin using all your fingers.

Step 2
Now push your fingers up to the corners of your mouth and massage this area.

Step 3
Move up to the nostrils and massage the corners.

Step 4
Massage along both sides of the nose to come to the eyebrows.
    Massage the inner ends of the eyebrows, then stroke your fingers along to the middle of each eyebrow.

Step 5
Now stroke straight up from the middle of the eyebrows to the hairline. Using a circular massaging motion, rub round the hairline down to the ears.

Step 6
Massage around the hairline behind the ears and then fold both the ears forward.

Step 7
Release the ears and continue massaging round the hairline at the back of the head.
    When the fingers meet in the middle, use the hands to massage the neck from the back round to the front. Repeat this process 6 times.

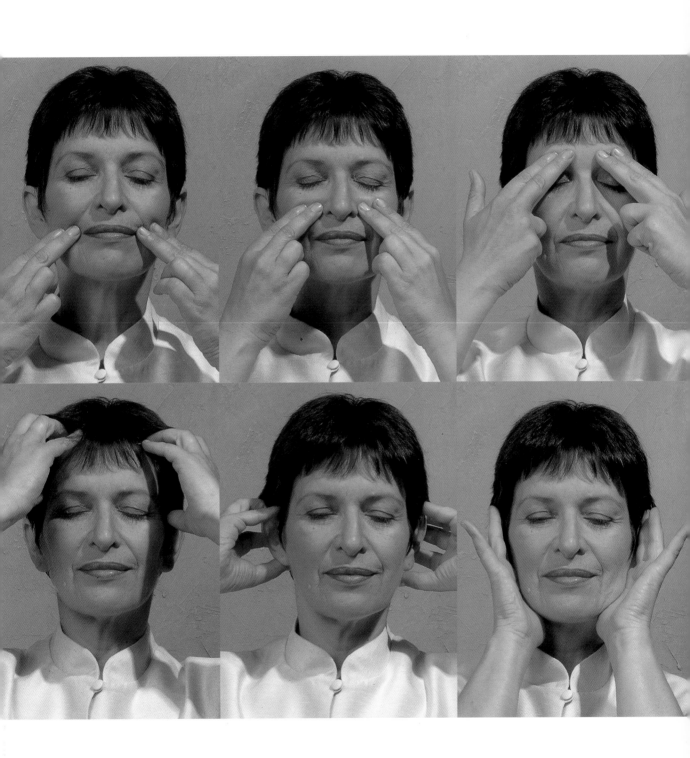

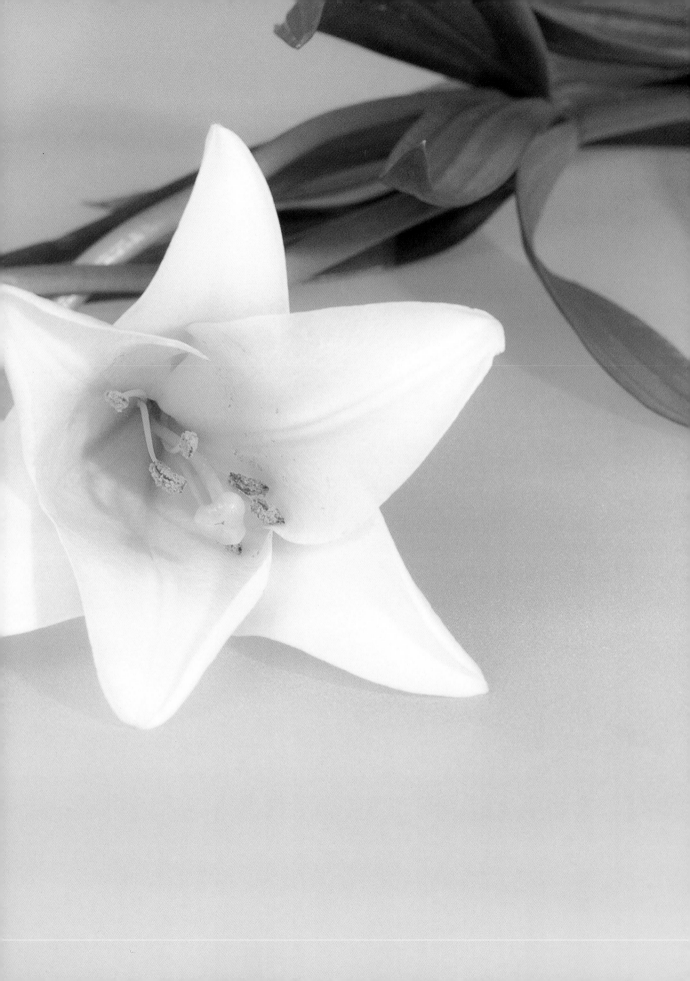

chi kung &
the ageing process

What is the essence of youth? It is health, energy and a positive mind. The young have an abundance of energy and they do not foresee a day when they will not be like that. They approach life as an adventure, eagerly anticipating every new experience and seeing nothing as impossible. If a child wants to be an astronaut, they see no reason why they shouldn't be. With age we begin to doubt that it is possible, but the child sees no obstacles. In the child's world, everything is possible. It is partly the loss of this belief that ages us as we surrender mentally, believing in the inevitable loss of physical and mental functions. Chi kung can add years to your life and life to your years, if you can believe once again that nothing is impossible.

combat ageing problems

The problems associated with ageing are diverse and there are few people, even the most healthy among us, who manage to go through their later years without experiencing any of them to some degree. It might be argued that many of these problems are largely preventable, yet most people, including the medical profession, accept them as inevitable facts of life. There are some problems associated with age that are now acknowledged to be lifestyle-related, such as heart attacks and strokes; these are not confined to people in the over-sixty age group, however, but are just more prevalent among the elderly.

Perhaps it is more correct to say that the real problems of ageing are not the dramatic events such as heart attacks, but the slow decline in body functions that seems to start in the mid-thirties and becomes more apparent after sixty. It is the failing eyesight, impaired hearing, pain and stiffness in the joints, rising or falling blood pressure, insomnia, dizziness and memory loss that are more defining of the problems of age. These are the changes that creep up on you slowly – instead of appearing suddenly and shocking you, they one day quietly come to your attention when you realize that you really can't climb that ladder any more, or that you can't hear what the person standing next to you is saying.

In the West we have no clear idea of how to prevent this decline or at least slow it down. Instead of tackling it in a systematic way, we ignore it, and decide that people over sixty, or even over fifty, are of no further use. In terms of energy, people in the older age groups cannot compete with the young, and energy of a certain type appears to be valued more, particularly by employers, than accumulated skills and knowledge. The fact that elderly people are perceived as having no contribution to make to society in itself contributes to the acceleration of physical and mental decline. Yet the term 'elderly' itself contains the word 'elder', a term that in less industrial societies, now and in the past, implies leadership and respect, whereas in the contemporary industrial society, the word 'elder' seems to be interpreted as 'burden'.

Chi kung offers a way by which elderly people can empower themselves again. Kenneth Cohen, in his book *The Way of Qigong* says that Chi kung cannot change your chronological age but it can change your *functional* age, and there are many reports of men and women over sixty who practise Chi kung and have the health and vitality of a person half their age. The efficacy of Chi kung is also demonstrated by the number of Chi kung masters who live to well over a hundred, although as one book by a Chi kung teacher points out, longevity is only desirable if it increases

the period of youthfulness, not that of old age. That is precisely what Chi kung can do.

Of course, Chi kung will only work effectively if it is practised regularly. For older people, the advantage of Chi kung is that it does not require a lot of physical exertion, and the exercises can be done lying down or sitting as well as standing up, so even those with limited physical function can use it to improve their lives. Also, while it can be practised alone, working together regularly in a group, as discussed before, has many advantages. For the elderly, the social benefits of attending a class cannot be underestimated as they are among the most isolated and lonely in our society.

how chi kung helps

How does Chi kung affect the ageing process? The essence of youth is characterized by health – physical and emotional well-being – and vitality – the energy for work and play. These are maintained by eating and sleeping well, being calm mentally and enjoying work, leisure time and sexual relations. If we maintain these throughout life, then we maintain health and vitality. But we tend not to do that. We particularly do not keep our minds calm and positive, as we usually allow stress to take over. Keeping the mind calm and positive is the key, as the mind leads the body.

Chi kung practice begins by building our innate biological energy, or *jing*, and one of our first responses is an improvement in appetite. This is important for older people, who often have a poor appetite; as food is one of our most important sources of energy, it is obvious that eating more and eating more healthily will increase the energy available to us. The Chi kung abdominal breathing technique (see page 48) also draws more energy into the body.

Chi kung also induces better-quality sleep, which helps to maintain the store of energy, and encourages suppleness in the spine so that *chi* energy can circulate freely to all parts of the body. These simple activities – eating, breathing and sleeping – are the keys to preserving the health and vitality of youth, which can be maintained throughout life, or at least improved, by Chi kung exercises.

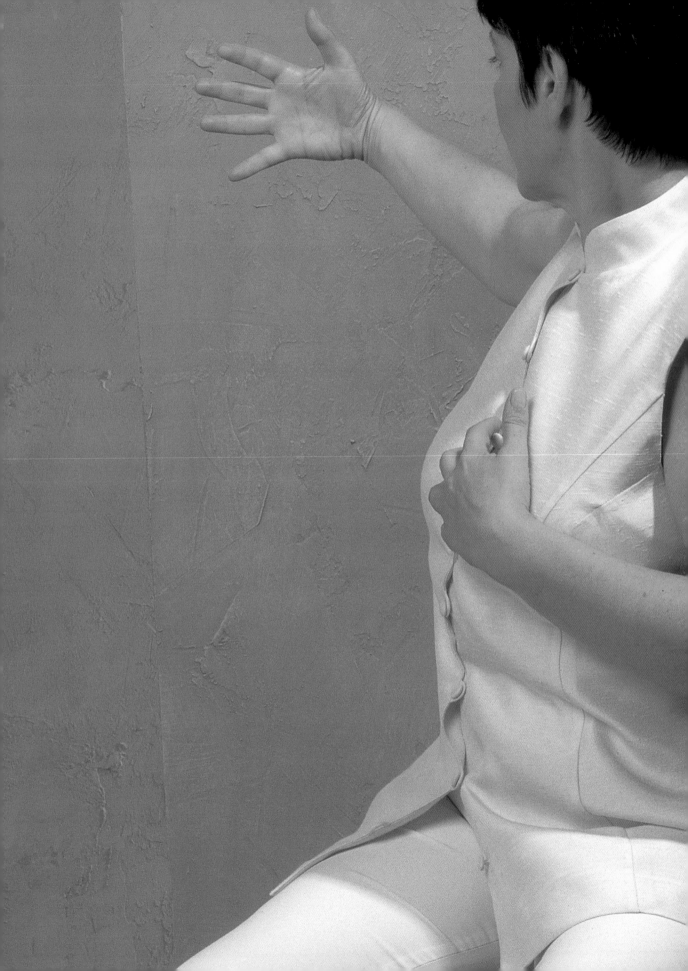

arthritis

Arthritis is defined as inflammation of the tissues of the joints. The two most common forms are osteoarthritis and rheumatoid arthritis. Osteoarthritis usually occurs in the knees, hips, neck, spine, fingers and thumbs. It is character-ized by stiffness and pain in the joints and 'creaking', which indicates that the joint cartilage has been worn away. Sufferers may also experience acute attacks of pain from swelling and inflammation of the joints, due to inflammation of the membranes surrounding the joints.

Rheumatoid arthritis is a condition in which the joints become inflamed and painful. Unlike osteoarthritis, it can make a person feel generally unwell, in addition to suffering pain and stiffness in the affected joints.

Both conditions are more common in women than in men, and while they are primarily associated with the ageing process, rheumatoid arthritis can start in the thirties and is more common in women over the age of 55 years.

Orthodox treatment for arthritis usually involves the use of painkillers and anti-inflammatory drugs in various forms along with physiotherapy, while people with advanced osteoarthritis may require joint-replacement surgery. In terms of non-orthodox treatment, arthritis is a condition that responds well to acupuncture, particularly for relief of the debilitating pain associated with it.

Chi kung is primarily used to prevent problems such as arthritis, but if you are already suffering from the condition, it can be used to relieve the symptoms. However, you should take care not to do exercises that overstrain the affected joints. In Chi kung the joints are considered to be the gate-ways that allow the energy to flow around the body, so con-sciously relaxing them all will promote a better flow. Even if you are not mobile, you can still be aware of your joints while sitting or lying down and can use your mind power to release the tension from them. The 'perfumed' Chi kung hand exercises (see pages 105–107) given in the section on using Chi kung at work are useful for pain in the wrist and hand joints, as are the Opening and closing the *chi* exercises (see page 50) in the daily routine and the Golden Cord, which is a revitalizing exercise (see page 114).

The Archer exercise is for opening the chest area and relaxing and releasing the shoulders, wrists and hands. It is also an excellent exercise for repetitive strain injury (RSI), which is caused by activities such as prolonged keyboard use and can affect the hands, wrists, arms, neck, shoulders and back.

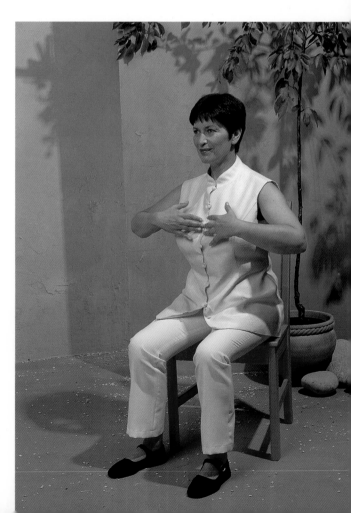

the archer

Step 1

Adopt a comfortable sitting posture with support for your back if you have spine or hip problems. Place both hands on your chest, with the elbows open and the tips of the middle fingers touching in the centre of your chest.

Step 2

Breathe in and stretch your right hand out to the right side. Keep your elbows relaxed and slightly rounded. Your hand should also be relaxed, with the fingers curling slightly inwards and the palm facing forwards.

Step 3

Keeping your attention on your palm, stretch your arm out and behind you. Repeat this on the other side. Alternatively, as you stretch your arm behind you, push your wrist and fingers backwards while making a loose fist with your other hand and pulling the arm out to the side, as if you were about to shoot an arrow from a bow. This is a more aggressive way of stretching the total nerve root, while the first version embodies the soft and flowing movements of Chi kung.

Another way to keep your hands supple and both prevent or alleviate arthritis is to rest your wrists on a table or on your knees and move your fingers as if playing the piano. This is also good for keyboard operators.

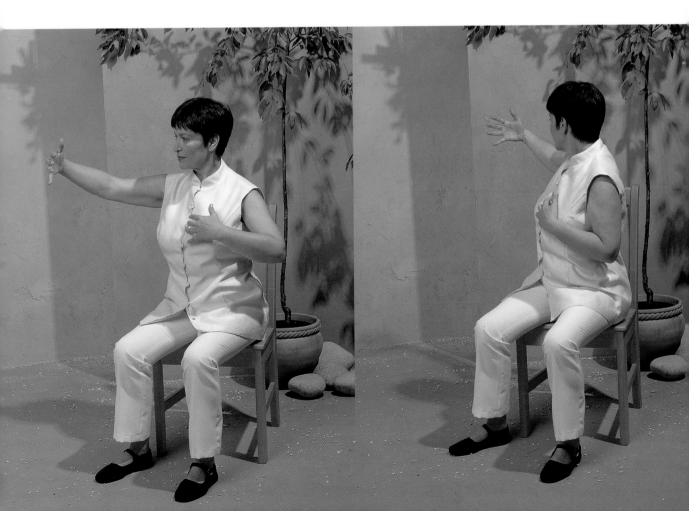

dizziness

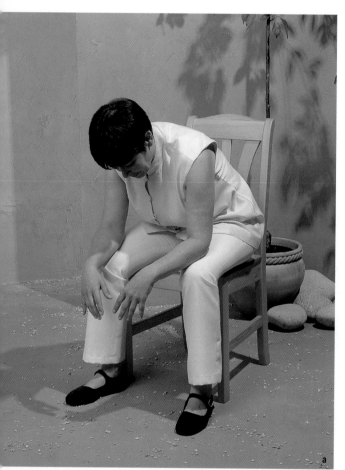

Dizziness does not affect only elderly people and the exercises recommended here can be used by anyone who is prone to dizzy spells. However, dizziness is of greater concern among the elderly because of its possible consequences; for example, it can lead to falls that may have serious results such as fractures, or unconsciousness from hitting the head when falling.

There are many causes of dizziness, and if you experience the feeling frequently you should consult a doctor first before attempting to resolve the problem yourself. Dizziness can be caused by the sympathetic nervous system's reaction to stress. It can also be a failure in the body's homeostatic system. This is the self-healing mechanism within the body that works to rectify health problems and achieve balance. However, this mechanism can be upset by stress, drugs, diet and other environmental factors.

Dizziness is also a symptom of Menière's disease, which is a condition of the ears, and some women may experience it as a secondary symptom of the menopause. It is also associated with problems of the circulatory system such as high or low blood pressure.

Dizziness can also be caused by over-practising Chi kung. This is often due to too much nervous energy in the head or lack of oxygen from over-breathing. There is a belief in classical Chi kung that the postures need to be correct for the *chi* to flow smoothly. If the *chi* cannot flow smoothly then the mind cannot focus properly, and if the mind cannot concentrate then the *chi* becomes blocked. This blockage can manifest as dizziness and a feeling of nausea.

treating dizziness

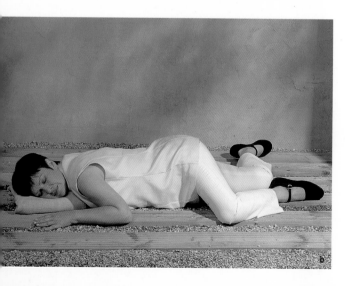

The solution to the onset of dizziness associated with Chi kung practice is to stop immediately and sit down with the feet firmly connected to the floor (see above left). If the dizziness is caused by over-breathing it is better to lie down. However, if you experience nausea as well do not lie down flat on your back.

Adopting the 'recovery position' will help overcome dizziness whatever its cause (see left). It is also a useful first-aid technique. Lie on one side, with your knees bent and apart and your head on a pillow. Place one arm on the floor behind your back with the uppermost arm bent comfortably in front of your face. If you have been doing a visualization lying on the floor, it is a good idea to roll into this position first before getting up off the floor, as it will prevent you from feeling light-headed when you get up.

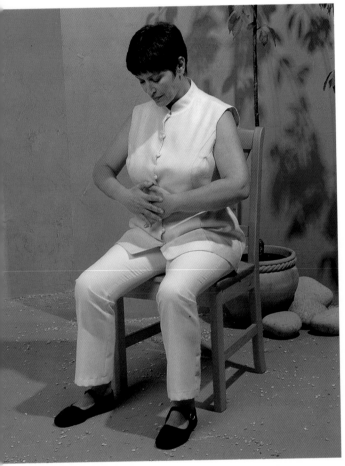
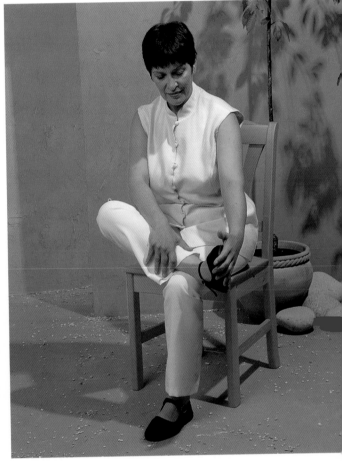

Step 1

Assume a sitting position and bring your focus down to *Dantian*, drawing the energy there in your mind. Calm your breathing, but keep it natural and try to lengthen the out-breath. Focus your mind on the kidneys and, while doing so, place your hands over each other with the palms facing the navel, and massage the area in a circular motion 36 times clockwise and 36 times anti-clockwise. This will bring the energy to the centre and help you to feel centred.

Step 2

Place the *Laogong* points in the centre of the palms over the kidney points on the soles of the feet and rub them.

hypertension

Hypertension, or high blood pressure as it is more commonly known, is increasingly common. The term 'blood pressure' refers to the force and volume of blood pumped by the heart on each beat and to the resistance to that force and volume by the larger blood vessels. In technical terms, one is the systolic pressure and the other is diastolic pressure. Blood pressure is defined as being high when there is a sustained rise above the accepted normal levels. Hypertension tends not to cause symptoms, and is therefore often found only during routine health screens. It is therefore important to ensure that you have your blood pressure checked regularly since hypertension leads to stroke and heart disease.

The majority of cases of hypertension have no precise underlying cause, although a small proportion are due to kidney disease, pregnancy and the use of drugs such as the contraceptive pill and steroids. For most cases, it is generally a result of lifestyle factors such as obesity, alcohol intake and stress. Methods of treatment recommended by orthodox

practitioners as well as many complementary therapies involve a change in lifestyle, with particular emphasis on diet, exercise and relaxtion techniques. These alone can bring down blood pressure in many people without the need for any drug intervention.

Increasing evidence that psychological factors, such as stress, play a significant part in hypertension has led to recognition of the importance of methods that teach a person who suffers from high blood pressure how to relax mentally as well as physically.

If stress factors combined with a poor lifestyle are the main contributing factors to hypertension, then the problem is easily reversed. This is not quite the case for people who have an inherited disposition towards the condition, although Chi kung, as a preventive health measure, can help them, too. However, even Chi kung will not cure hypertension if lifestyle factors such as overeating or too much salt in the diet are not rectified.

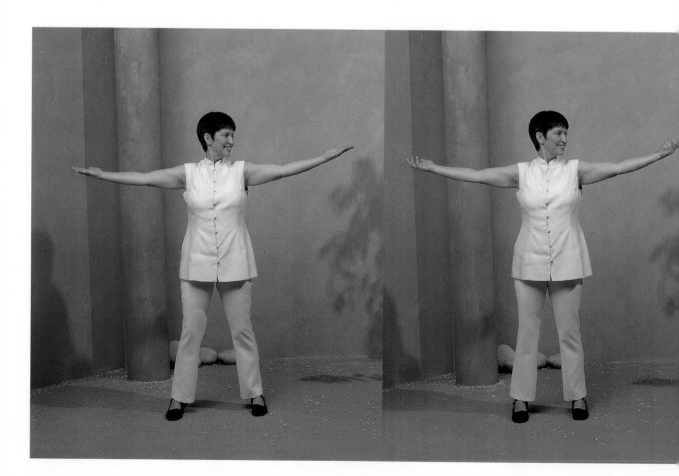

relieving hypertension

The following two exercises can help to relieve hypertension. The first exercise (not shown) is for mental relaxation and can be done lying down or sitting. First imagine that warm water is flowing from the top of your head down the front of the body to your feet. Then imagine that the water is flowing from the top of the head down your back and then that it is flowing down the sides of the body. Repeat this, following the three routes, for at least 20 minutes. Then, while in the Chi kung standing position

(see page 47), sway gently from side to side and imagine the warm water flowing down your body and out through the soles of your feet. Keep repeating this and intentionally take your awareness down to your fingertips and toes, drawing the energy down.

Step 1
Stand in the Chi kung posture with your hands at your sides. Turn the palms outwards and raise your arms up. At the same time rise up a little on your toes.

Step 2
When you have brought your arms to shoulder height, with the palms facing up, curl each finger, one by one, into the palm of your hand so they cover the *Laogong* points and make a fist.

Step 3
Rotate your wrists to turn the fists over. Stretch your arms and raise your fists from the wrist.

Step 4
Now release your fingers and bring your hands down.

Step 5
Repeat steps 1–4, four to six times. Finish by opening your legs and, with knees and elbows bent, shake out your hands.

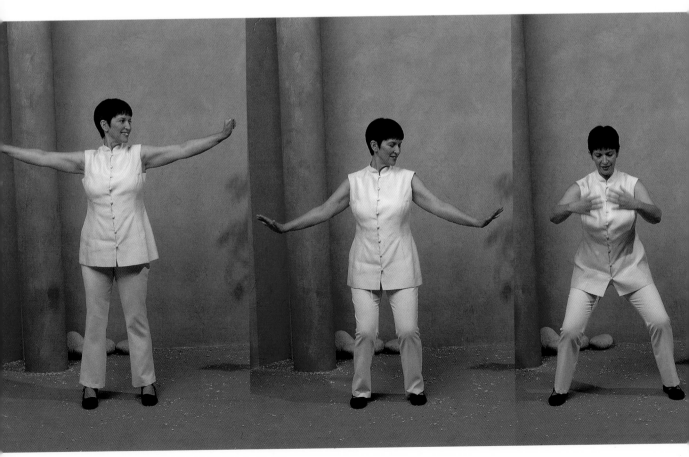

chi kung in the workplace

Stress and work are two words that unfortunately seem to go together. Increasingly, if you ask someone how their life is going they will reply that they are stressed by their work. It is not surprising then that work stress is thought to be the primary cause of physical and mental illness in Western society. The potential cost of this stress to the individual is premature death, while the cost to employers is a financial one, through loss of productivity. What is needed is a simple, cost-effective method of eliminating negative stress from the workplace for the benefit of everyone there.

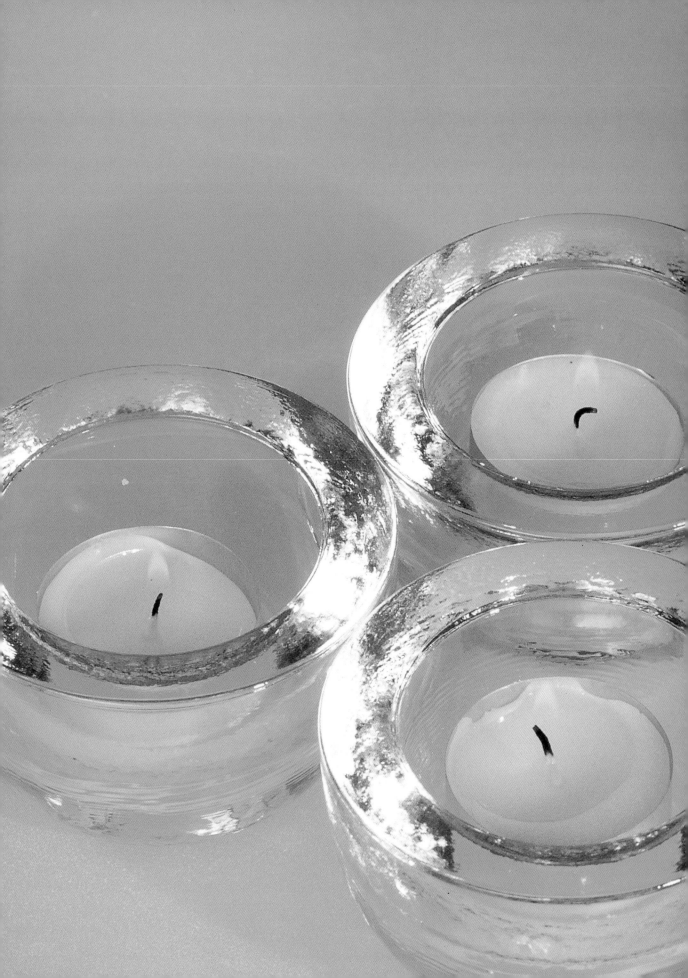

the causes of physical stress at work

Work stress originates from three potential sources:

• individual circumstance
• work environment
• organizational structure

The first is beyond the control of the employer and includes individual personality and domestic circumstances. It is impossible for most people to separate such stress from their work life and 'leave it at home'. When personal life stresses impinge on work, they will be compounded by stress at work and the vicious cycle of stress becomes harder to break. Employers are now recognizing that it is unrealistic to expect workers with problems in their personal lives to perform at full capacity, and are increasingly providing confidential counselling services and other such help for their workers.

The environmental source of stress is not only the work environment, but also aspects outside the employer's control, such as national economic and political uncertainty and the perception that society and technology are changing at an ever-faster pace. Technology is a key source of stress: in the post-industrial society mechanization has increasingly taken over from human input, particularly since the widespread use of computers. The significance of this in terms of stress is that the speed of work has increased and humans are being required to keep up with the speed of machinery. Also, the loss of autonomy or personal control over work processes, a problem once associated with production-line work, has now spread into office-based work.

Organizational factors causing stress include work over-load, career blocks and dysfunctional working relationships, particularly between managerial staff and the workforce. These are the responsibility of employers and can only be controlled by them. Businesses demand ever higher efficiency and speedier production and the stress this induces in workers may result in weakened immune function, an increase in viral disorders and a weakened nervous system, sometimes resulting in nervous breakdown.

We need to work for practical reasons and perhaps, more importantly, to feel fulfilled through using our individual abilities, but work should not make us sick. While certain factors within the workplace can be controlled only by the employer, the employee can also take steps to control work stress, first by ensuring that employers are aware of the stress factors

and second, by taking steps to control their own response to stress – otherwise known as stress management. Such is the problem that employers are bringing in stress management consultants to train staff in techniques for alleviating stress. Research shows that stress management involves training in relaxation techniques, maintenance of physical fitness and teaching individuals how to find time for themselves. This last issue is a significant one for people who are employed in the home and are often ignored in discussions about work – parents or carers have difficulty finding time for themselves as there are no controls over their working day, which in some cases can be nearly 24 hours. In cases other than that of home-workers, one solution is for employers to ensure that workers systematically take time out from work for self-renewal, which in the long term would benefit both parties.

The most common signals of stress at work are:

• persistent fatigue
• irritability
• poor concentration

A host of physical and mental signals indicate stress: head-aches, muscle tension in the neck and shoulders, palpitations, excessive sweating, dizziness and increased smoking or drinking are just a few of the signs. Psychologically, the symptoms are a tendency to worry, feelings of apprehension or impending doom, being rude and irritable and losing interest in hobbies outside work and in the job itself. When you recognize these signs and, most importantly, accept that you are not the only one suffering in this way, you can start taking steps to solve the problem. The exercises and suggestions in this section are to help you do this. They are simple activities that you can do every day while at work. A relaxing visualization need take only a few minutes and can be done at your desk or at a nearby park at lunchtime. Exercises to relieve the strain of using a keyboard are also unobtrusive.

Chi kung has a lot to offer in terms of work stress relief, providing mental relaxation and preventing the physical problems caused by working at a computer for long periods and using poorly designed office furniture. When you, and hopefully your colleagues, experience the benefits of Chi kung, perhaps you can persuade your employer to provide a weekly class and the time and space for everyone to practise.

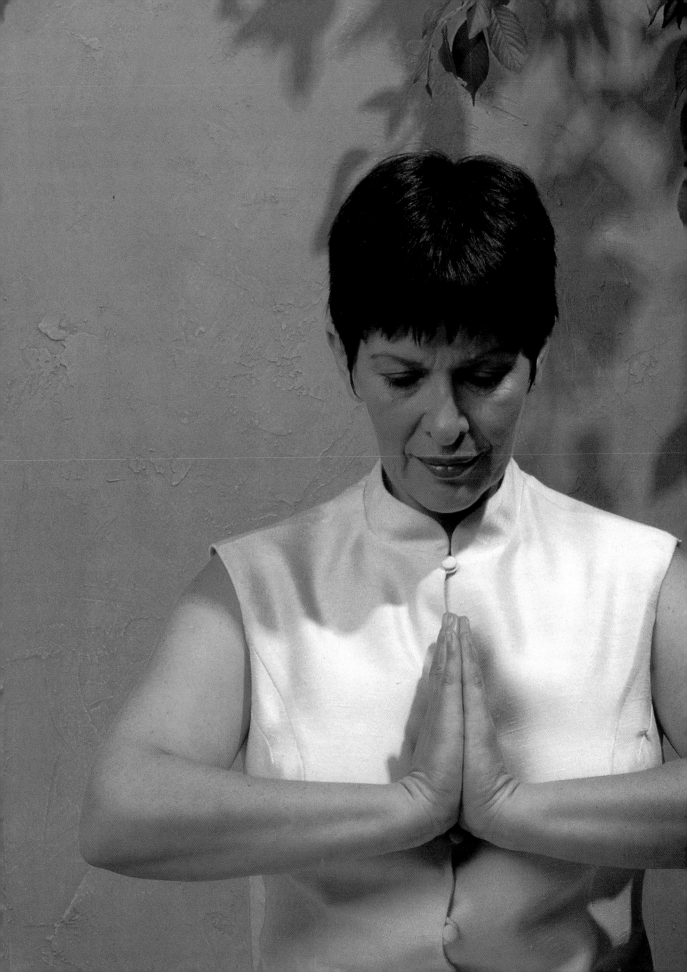

dealing with stress

Here are some simple suggestions to make your work life physically and mentally more comfortable and enjoyable. Not all of them are Chi kung as such, but they are definitely in the spirit of Chi kung as they encourage mental calm and the release of energy.

Look first of all at the environment in which you work. You should, of course, have an appropriate style of office chair, a proper desk and workspace and a screen for your computer monitor, if you use one, to cut out the glare from the screen. Try to make your workspace as attractive as possible within the allowed limits. Plants in particular are good for this as they radiate *chi* energy. If you like crystals, you could place one or two on your computer as they are thought to reduce the amount of electro-magnetic radiation coming from the computer.

Make sure that your workspace is well lit and, if possible, do not sit facing a wall or have your back to the office door. The best position is to be near a window, and the most comfortable offices have plenty of windows and natural light. I once worked in a basement office that had only one window and there was never enough natural light for the artificial lights to be turned off. After a while I realized that everyone in that office was always sick, including myself. I concluded that this was the result of being both in a basement and always in artificial light, and I certainly believed in 'sick building syndrome' after that experience. Sick building syndrome refers to a theory that says some buildings are constructed in a way that promotes ill health in the people who live or work in them.

The following exercises will help you to link gentle physical movement with inner relaxation and breathing techniques to allow your sympathetic nervous system to rest.

correct sitting posture

Every time you sit down at your desk, take a few minutes and adjust yourself into the Chi kung sitting posture (see page 46). Make sure your chair is at the right height so that you can sit with both your feet comfortably on the floor. It is not good to sit for long periods with your legs crossed, so try to avoid that as well. In the Chi kung sitting posture, your bottom should be towards the front of the chair so that your *Huiyin* point or perineum is on the edge of the chair. Visualize a golden cord attached to the *Baihui* point on your crown pulling your head up into the sky. Both your feet should be flat on the floor so that the kidney points have good contact with it, and you should be able to feel your weight in the soles of your feet.

taking a break

When you are sitting at your desk, take a complete break from your computer by switching it off. The constant noise it makes, the screen glare and the electro-magnetic radiation are all irritants, even when you are not working on the computer. Do this whenever you can, particularly if you have lunch at your desk.

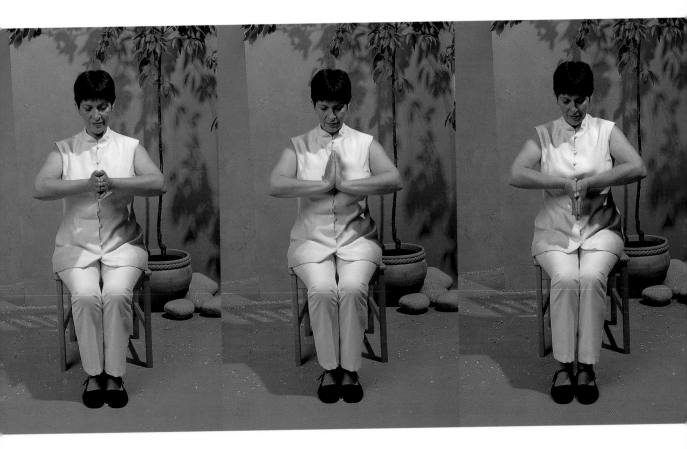

peacock nodding

This and the following exercises are known as 'perfumed Chi kung', because when the complete routine is practised it is said that there is a beautiful smell in the air.

Step 1
Hold your hands together at chest level in the normal praying position, but with your fingers pointing away from you, instead of upwards, and your elbows opened at your sides.

Step 2
Tap your chest by bending your wrists up so that your thumbs hit the point in the middle of your sternum.

Step 3
Now bend your wrists down so that your little fingers knock against the stomach. Repeat this up/down movement at least 12 times. After you have practised it for a few days you can build it up to 24 and then to 36 times.

dragon wagging tail

Step 1
Start as for the Peacock Nodding exercise by placing your hands together at chest level, again with your fingers pointing away from you, but this time with fingers spread and keeping your elbows wide open.

Step 2
Now use your left hand to push your right wrist so that it bends back and the fingers are pointing to the right.

Step 3
Now switch over so that the right wrist pushes the left wrist back, and the fingers are now pointing left. Repeat this 12 times at first and then build up to 24 and then to 36 repetitions.

releasing tension

Rest your wrists on your desk, on the back of a chair (see right), or on your knees. As you breathe out, stretch your fingers away from you. Keep stretching them and visualize all toxins and blockages in your circulatory system leaving your body on every out-breath. This is an exercise that you can practise frequently throughout the day.

This tension-releasing exercise is particularly good for people who drive all day, such as bus drivers and long-distance lorry drivers. If you are confined in a car for long periods of time you can do the exercise while at traffic lights or when you are stuck in a traffic jam. Stretching the fingers away from you releases all the 'fight or flight' in your muscles. Also, if you visualize the release of toxins, or of anger and other pent-up feelings, the combination of exercise with visualization is a form of Chi kung.

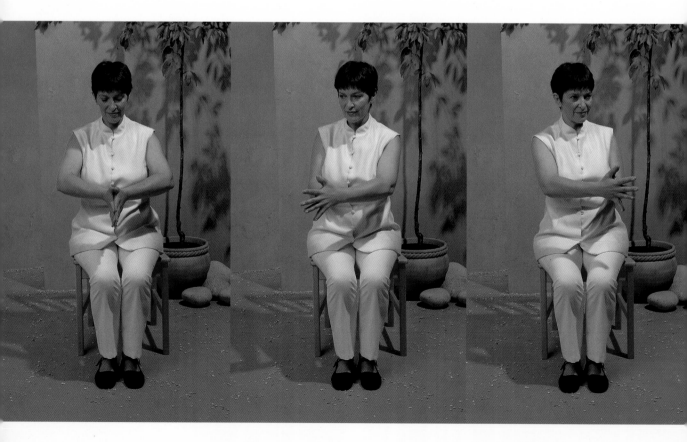

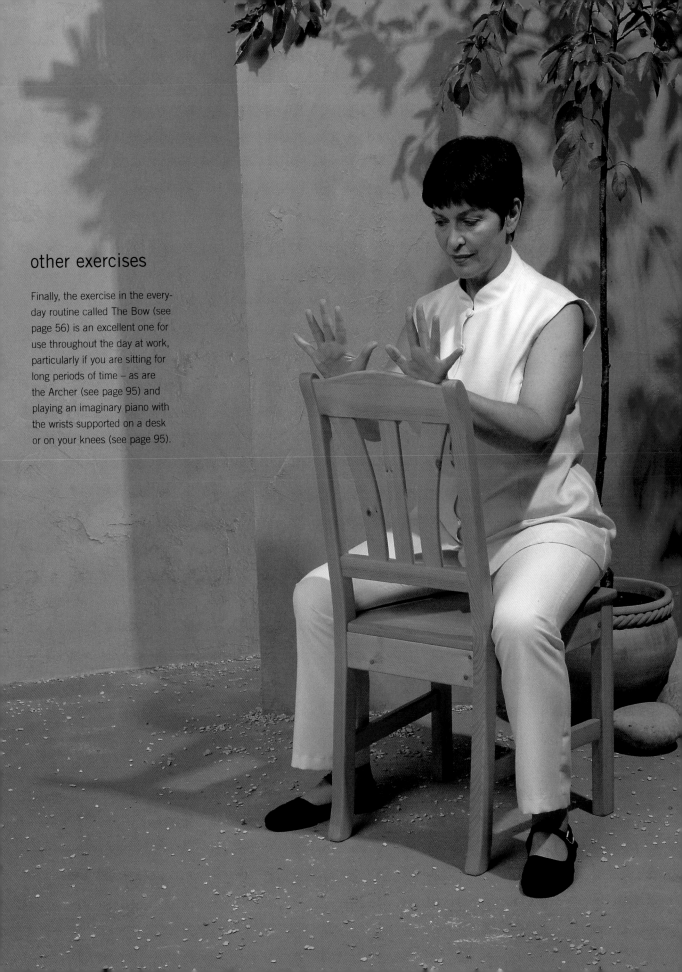

other exercises

Finally, the exercise in the every-day routine called The Bow (see page 56) is an excellent one for use throughout the day at work, particularly if you are sitting for long periods of time – as are the Archer (see page 95) and playing an imaginary piano with the wrists supported on a desk or on your knees (see page 95).

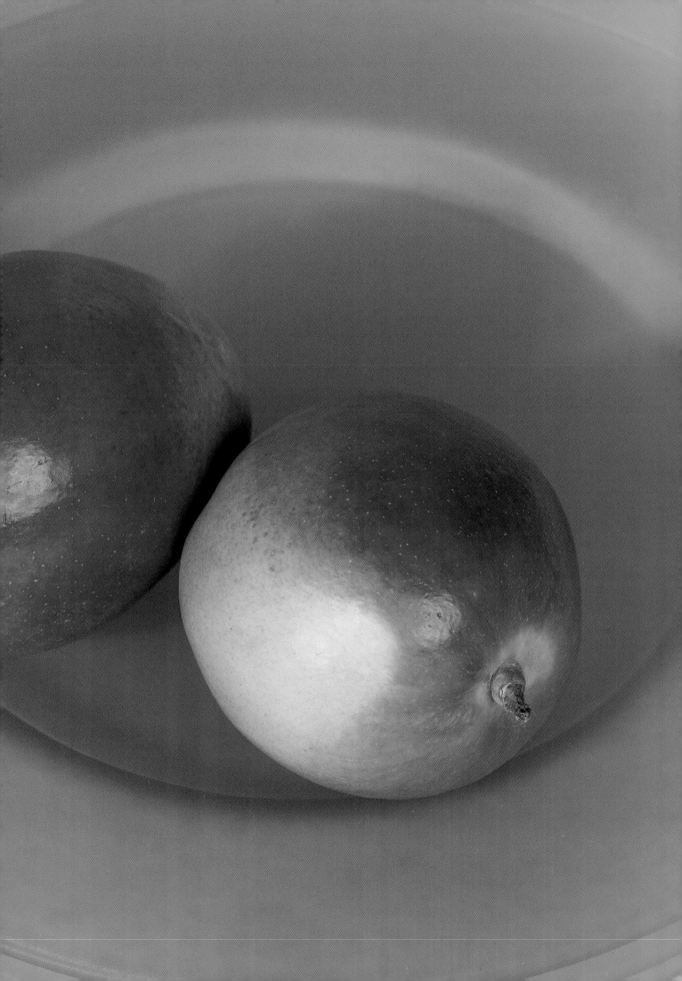

chi kung for common ailments

In the *Yellow Emperor's Classic of Internal Medicine* it says that 'mediocre medicine cures disease: superior medicine prevents it'. Accordingly, Chinese medical philosophy has always emphasized the importance of prevention over cure. The benefit of Chi kung is that, while it is primarily seen as a superior method of preventing ill health, when you practise it you can both prevent and cure at the same time.

When we are in perfect health our bodies will easily cope with an invasion of cold germs or 'flu virus. If it is functioning well, the body will also deal with toxins and with stress. However, this is an ideal condition which few of us, it seems, enjoy. With Chi kung we can prevent both serious diseases and minor ailments – and we can cure them as well.

external & internal causes of ailments

According to Chinese medical philosophy, ailments have external causes, which have their sources in nature and the man-made environment, and internal causes that are emotional. Avoiding excesses of any of these promotes balance and therefore good health.

external causes

Wind – this represents both movement and change. It is thought to invade the body, which is why people are cautioned not to practise Chi kung outside when it is windy. When wind is combined with cold, you are more likely to catch colds and 'flu, and in Chinese thinking the wind is most harmful in spring.

Cold – this limits movement and can therefore lead to stagnation of energy. It is most likely to affect the lungs, while cold in the stomach can result in vomiting and diarrhoea.

Fire/heat – typically an excess of this is associated with fevers, inflammation and constipation. It may also manifest as irritability and lack of concentration. Heat in summer should also be avoided in excess as it results in heatstroke and dehydration.

Dryness – this is similar to fire but in addition it dries up the body fluids. Therefore constipation is also associated with this element, as is dry skin, cracked lips and dry coughs.

Damp – this is associated with heaviness and typical symptoms resulting from an excess of it are lethargy, swollen joints and headaches.

internal causes

Joy – according to the Chinese, an excess of joy can damage the heart and cause insomnia, heart palpitations and over-excitement.

Anger – the emotions associated with anger, which can range from rage to resentment, injure the liver and cause high blood pressure, headaches and stomach-related illnesses.

Sadness – this affects the lungs and heart and can cause tiredness and weaken the immune system.

Pensiveness – too much thought or intellectual work affects the spleen and can cause loss of appetite and anaemia.

Fear – this affects the kidneys and as a result can reduce fertility and the sexual appetite as well as reducing resistance to infection.

Shock – the heart and the kidneys are most affected by this, with palpitations and insomnia being typical reactions.

While these reflect an Oriental system of thought, similar observations are made within our own culture – but we don't integrate them into our medical system. We are aware that a damp atmosphere causes us to feel lethargic and prone to headaches, but we do not suggest to the doctor that damp is the cause of our problem, but put it down to something that seems to us more rational. However, if we say that we feel 'a bit under the weather', we would be right. The Chinese system is primarily concerned with balance and regularity – 'everything in moderation' is the key to it – and by observing this guideline you can help yourself to avoid both major and minor ailments.

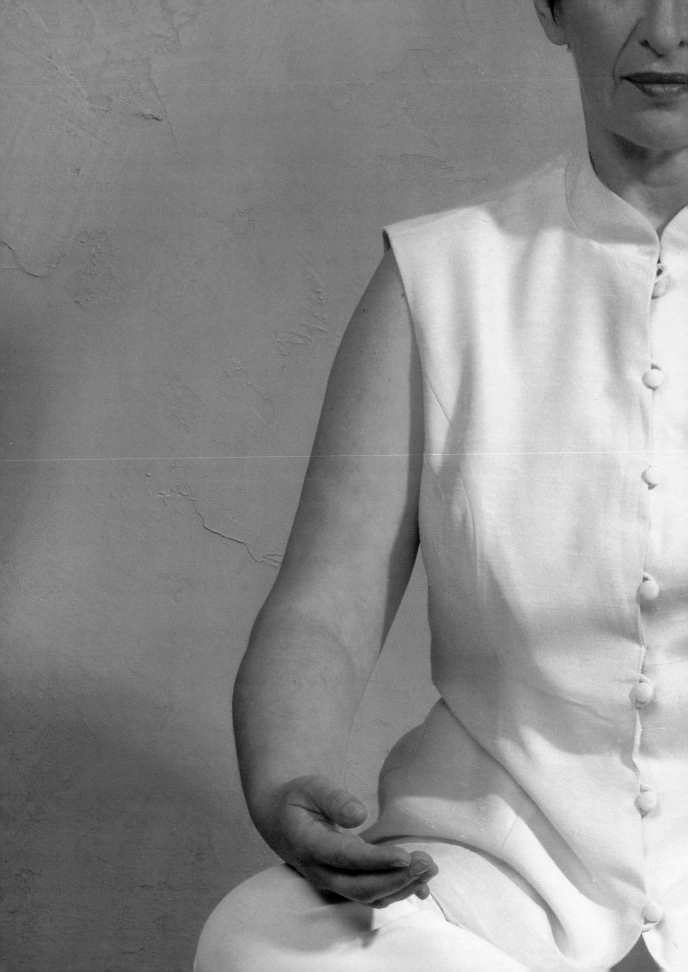

treatments for common ailments or injuries

What follows is a number of specially selected exercises for common problems. They can form part of your daily Chi kung routine or they can be used only when the need arises. You can also use the exercises in conjunction with aromatherapy oils, homeopathy, Bach flowers and other forms of treatment to speed up the healing process.

eye rolls

This exercise is a good follow-up to the eye-strengthening exercise (see right). Do not move your head while doing it, and perform the movements slowly and deliberately. Stop between each movement and look straight ahead. It takes approximately 10 minutes to do this exercise slowly.

1 Look straight ahead.
2 Look up at the ceiling.
3 Look down at the ground.
4 Look to the left.
5 Look to the right.
6 Look up at a slant to both
   left and right.
7 Rotate the eyes clockwise.
8 Rotate the eyes anti-clockwise.

eye strengthening exercise

In Chinese medicine it is believed that the eyes are connected with the liver and that problems with the liver will result in problems with the eyes and vice versa. Doing this eye exercise will therefore strengthen both the eyes and the liver and help to prevent cataracts and other conditions such as eyestrain and short-sightedness. In this exercise you will be putting pressure on the meridian points that lie on the bone around the eye, and in doing so stimulating the energy and breaking up any energy blocks.

Step 1
Begin by pressing with your thumbs or middle finger on the point at the inner end of each eyebrow. Exert as much direct pressure as you can for about 10 seconds. Then rub the points. If you feel pain it means there is some weakness here.

Now move your thumbs or fingers to the next point, in the middle of the eye socket below the eye, and again exert pressure on them for 10 seconds, followed by rubbing the points.

Step 2
The next point at which to apply pressure is on the bottom of the eye socket again, near the outside corner of the eye. Follow the same procedure as for Step 1.

Step 3
Now move your fingers to just below the outer end of the eyebrow and press there.

Step 4
The last point is on the outer edge of the eye socket as it meets the temple – just beyond the outer edge of the eyebrows. Follow the same procedure as before. When you have completed this sequence, repeat it three more times.

Step 5
When you have done this rub round the eye socket in a circular motion starting at the inner corner of the eye, rubbing up the bridge of the nose, over the eyebrows and then from the inner corner to the outer along the lower edge of the eye socket. Don't push skin from the outer corner to the inner – it will cause wrinkles.

Step 6
Finish by rubbing your hands together vigorously and placing your palms over your eyes.

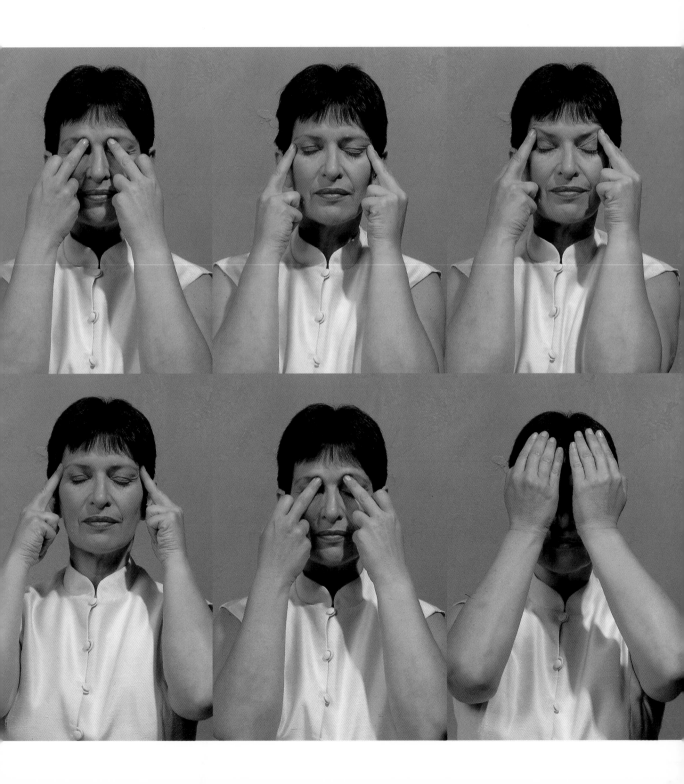

beating an energy slump

We all experience times when we seem to have no energy, so here are some simple ways to revive yourself during the day, whether you are at home or at work.

ear massage

In Chinese medicine the ear is believed to contain a micro-system of the whole body with each part of the ear relating to an internal organ or other body part. Massaging the ears is an easily accessible way of clearing stale toxins from the body. Alternatively, you can achieve the same effect by massaging the soles of your feet with the palms of your hands.

Step 1
Put your hands behind your ears and push your ears forwards to cover the ear hole. Repeat this 2–3 times.

Step 2
Massage the outer rim of each ear from top to bottom between your thumb and first finger.

Step 3
Massage your earlobe.

Step 4
With the index or middle finger rub around the inside of each ear, in the outer part at first.

Step 5
Then progress to the area around the eardrum, going over each part thoroughly.

Step 6
By now your ears should be feeling warm and tingly. Finish off by gently cupping your hands over your ears, then massage your neck with down-ward movements.

the golden cord

Stand or sit in the Chi kung posture, ensuring that the *Baihui* point on the crown of the head is directly in line with the *Huiyin* point at the perineum. Now imagine that you are suspended by a golden cord from the sky that is attached to the *Baihui* point. Feel your neck elongate, then your spine, until you feel taller. Breathe into the entire length of the spine. Breathe into each space between the vertebrae so that they feel open and elastic. Imagine that with each breath fresh oxygen is nourishing the spaces between the vertebrae. Pause between each breath and feel the blood and fluids around and through the spinal column. Do this until you feel refreshed by this simple stretch. Finish by rubbing your hands together and then rub your face, or any other parts of your body that need attention. Finally, shake your hands and feet.

arm swinging

This exercise will give you a quick charge of energy and will improve the circulation of blood and chi. This is also a very good exercise for the elderly. You can do the exercise for as long as you feel comfortable, but three minutes should be long enough for you to feel the effects.

Stand with your body relaxed in the Chi kung posture with the arms hanging naturally at the sides. Breathe naturally. Focusing on your feet, imagine that they are gripping the ground. Your toes will curl inwards and your heels will press into the ground, creating a feeling of sucking energy up through the kidney points.

Now swing your arms alter-nately to the front and back. Do not lift them too high at first, particularly if you have a shoul-der problem. Establish a flowing rhythm and, as you finish the exercise, gradually reduce the swing of your arm movements.

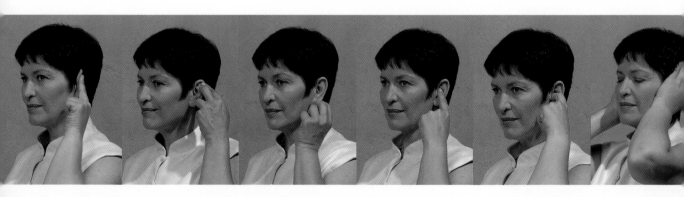

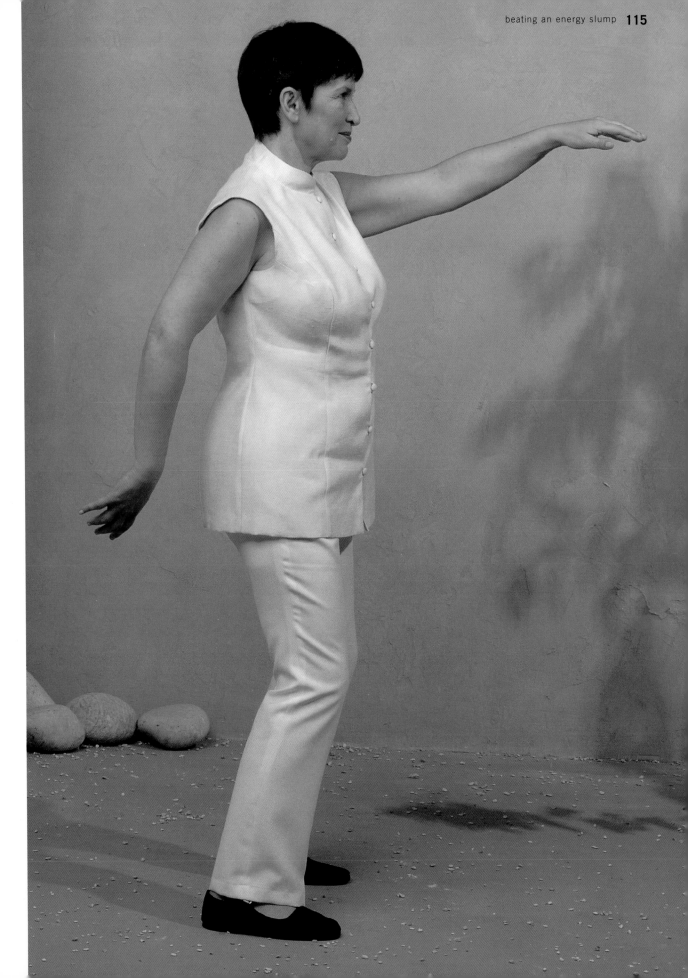

colds & 'flu

If you have a very severe cold or 'flu, the best thing is to rest and allow your body to start healing itself. When you are feeling better resume your Chi kung exercises, which will help to eliminate the lingering after-effects more quickly. Of course it is preferable not to get either a cold or 'flu in the first place, and hopefully you will find that by using Chi kung regularly your susceptibility to these will decrease. As part of the Chi kung preventive measures you should also keep warm in cold weather and never practise in cold and windy places, which allows the body to be invaded by external pollutants.

Cold and 'flu prevention is based on a strong immune system and getting rid of blocked energy. Two methods of doing this which have already been described involve releasing pathogenic *chi* using the technique in the warm-up exercises (see page 43), and practising the Eagle from the daily exercise routine (see page 54), which strengthens the immune system. Other preventive methods are:

• Doing the stomach massage, which is described in the section on dizziness (see page 96) and which will warm up the stomach

• Massaging the nostrils and face (see page 88) to clear blockages and help you to feel more clear-headed, 'huffing' the breath out of the nostrils as you do so

• Doing the Meridian Massage (see page 44)

• Having a full-body massage with oils, which will vitalize the skin and lungs

• Eating plenty of fresh fruit and vegetables and drinking plenty of water

• Avoiding smoking.

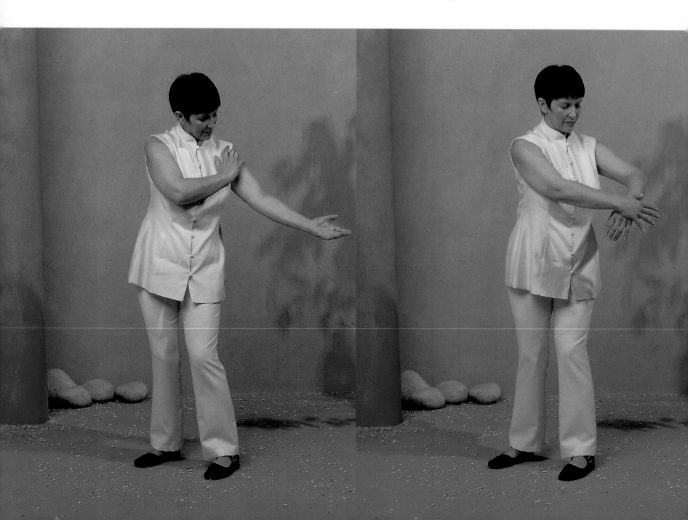

alternative meridian massage

This is a variation on the form described in the warm-ups (see page 44).

Step 1
Assume the standing Chi kung posture. With your right hand, stroke down the inside of your left arm, over your palm, to the tip of your little finger.

Step 2
Turning the left arm round, start to stroke up the back of the arm from the tip of your little finger.

Step 3
Continue stroking to the top of your arm.

Step 4
Continue to stroke up the neck, round the back of the ear, over the front of the ear, down the neck and down the inside of the arm to the little finger. Change over arms and repeat Steps 3 and 4. Do this 4–6 times.

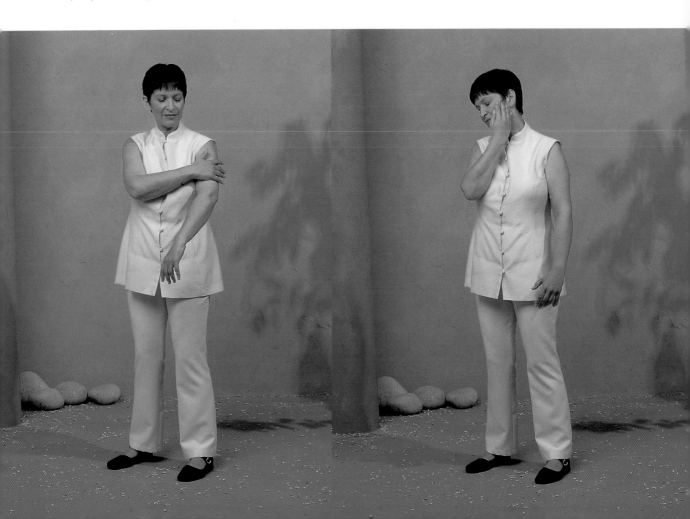

back & neck tension & headaches

Chronic pain is very difficult to bear and can be even more difficult to shift, and painkillers are often needed to break the cycle of pain. It is important to do this, because if you are crippled with pain you will not feel like tackling the problem with exercises. A build-up of tension in the back and in the neck can lead to headaches, and the exercises for loosening up muscular tension in the neck and shoulders, while not directly aimed at treating headaches, will help to prevent them.

There are precautions that we can take to prevent some of the tension build-up, however, a few of which have already been described in the section on using Chi kung in the workplace. Taking environmental measures, such as making sure that office and home furniture supports correct posture, is one approach. The other is to take time to practise correct posture and proper relaxation of the skeletal structure, particularly the spine. Even simply adopting the Chi kung standing or sitting position for a few minutes every day will help you to improve your general posture.

The following exercises will alleviate spine and neck problems and as a result help to prevent headaches caused by tension in these parts.

You should first loosen up the shoulder joints, using the Loosening Up exercise below. This method can also be used while working in a sedentary position to help release tension in the shoulders.

balancing energy

This exercise is good for people with problems of balance, and for preventing back pain. When you do the exercise, your waist and hip movements should be gentle rather than exaggerated. Be aware of changing the balance of weight from one foot to the other as your rotate your waist and hips.

Step 1

Stand naturally with the whole body relaxed and breathe naturally. Place your hands on your back over your kidneys, as if you were holding them.

Keeping both your legs straight, rotate your waist and hips in a clockwise direction. Do this 10 times.

Step 2

Then do the same exercise 10 times in an anti-clockwise direction. When you have finished, your back should feel warmer and more relaxed.

loosening up

With your hands loosely against your thighs, make several circles with alternate shoulders, first in a clockwise direction (towards your back) then in an anti-clockwise direction.

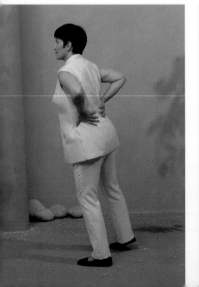
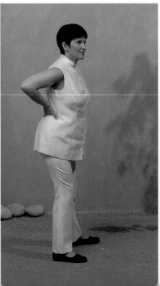

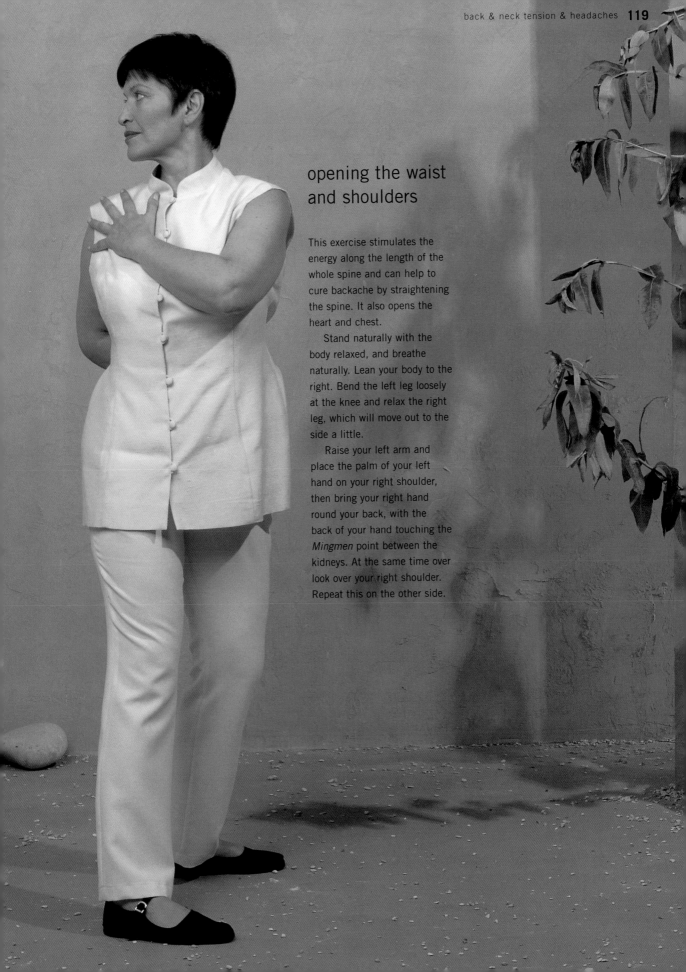

opening the waist and shoulders

This exercise stimulates the energy along the length of the whole spine and can help to cure backache by straightening the spine. It also opens the heart and chest.

Stand naturally with the body relaxed, and breathe naturally. Lean your body to the right. Bend the left leg loosely at the knee and relax the right leg, which will move out to the side a little.

Raise your left arm and place the palm of your left hand on your right shoulder, then bring your right hand round your back, with the back of your hand touching the *Mingmen* point between the kidneys. At the same time over look over your right shoulder. Repeat this on the other side.

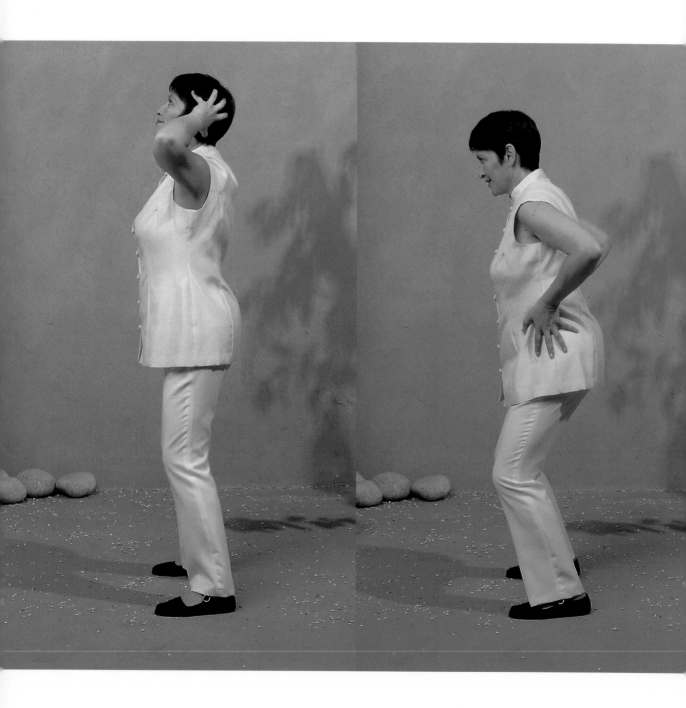

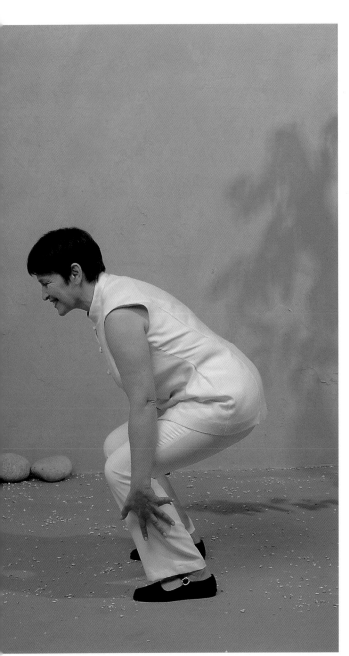

head massage for headaches

When massaging the head you are massaging the gall bladder meridian system. In TCM, the gall bladder is associated with the liver, which stores blood. When blood becomes blocked, clearing the gall bladder meridians clears the system of stagnation and is said to prevent headaches.

Step 1
Using your fingers, simply massage the head over the middle and down the back. Massage the sides and down the neck. You can do this when you are washing your hair as well as at other times.

Step 2
You can also extend this massage to other points on the gall bladder meridian at the sides of the waist.

Step 3
The lower legs are also worth massaging to treat headaches.

finding tranquillity

Finally, when you are too tired to do exercises, or you have difficulty sleeping or troubled dreams, or your head is over-heated from too much mental work, you can try this exercise, which according to the Shanghai Research Institute of Traditional Medicine is the best method of relaxing the entire nervous system. It is a form of meditative breathing based on the feminine Moon that cools and calms after the heat of the Sun. It is yin brought to balance yang.

Sit cross-legged, preferably on a small cushion so that you can maintain the natural curve of your spine and there is no strain on the ligaments around your pelvis. Sitting on a cushion also ensures that the pelvis is above the *Huiyin* point at the perineum. Let your shoulders be rounded and the chest drawn slightly in. Touch your palate with your tongue and allow your eyelids to droop and your hands to relax in your lap. Imagine that all your joints are open and that there is no tension in your muscles. You feel light and cheerful as you smile at all your internal organs.

Once you feel comfortable in this position, breathe out two or three long breaths, without breathing in. Let go of your internal organs and diaphragm. When you have breathed out as much as you can, your natural reflex will draw air in and fill up the abdomen without you consciously controlling it. Once the in-breath has finished you repeat the process.

When you feel completely comfortable with your breathing, let your eyes focus downwards at a 45 degree angle to a point just in front of your knees. As you become practised in the technique you will see various colours that will gradually fade to a misty white. Imagine the white light is the full Moon radiating its light all around you. You may feel as though you are in a peaceful place where the air is bright and clear, and where your body feels revived and your mind is free of worry and anxiety.

Immerse yourself in the light, saying silently to yourself, 'The light is me, I am the light.' As time passes you will feel one with the light, still and bright like it. You will feel clear like moonlight and you may even forget that you have a body.

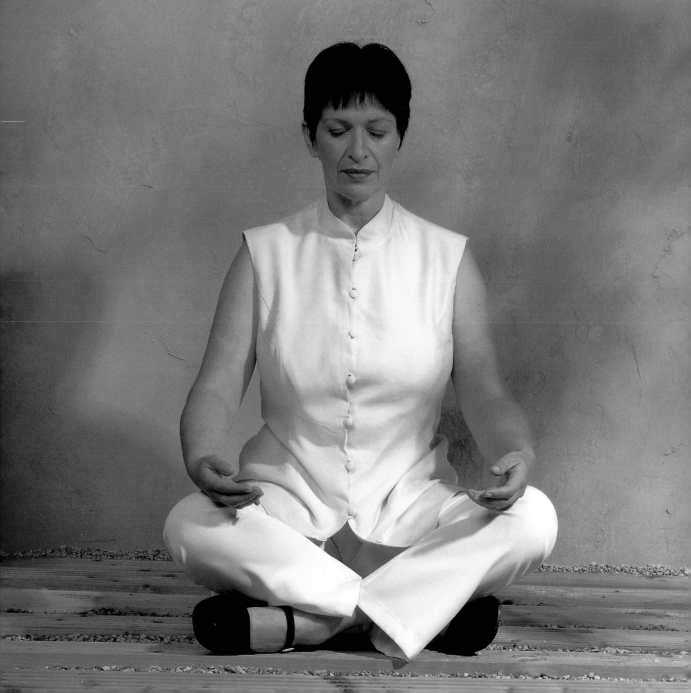

bibliography

MacRitchie, James *Chi Kung* Element Books, Dorset, 1993

Wong, Lydia *Qinetics* video and book available from
P. Wong, 14 Hows Close, Uxbridge, Middx UB8 2AS

Cohen, Kenneth S. *The Way of Qigong* Bantam Books,
London, 1997

Wong Kiew Kit *The Art of Chi Kung – making the most of
your vital energy* Element Books, Dorset, 1993

Alton, John *Living Qigong – the Chinese way to good health
and long life* Shambala, Boston, 1997

Tse, Michael *Qigong for Health and Vitality* Tse Qigong
Centre, PO Box 116, Manchester M20 3YN

Yuefang, Chen *Chinese Qigong Essentials* New World Press,
Beijing, 1996

Chia, Mantak *Cultivating Female Sexual Energy* Healing Tao
Books, New York, 1986

Chia, Mantak *Chi Self-Massage – the Taoist way to
rejuvenation* Healing Tao Books, New York, 1986

Quinn, Khaleghl *Chi Kung – reclaim your power*
Thorsons, London, 1991

Lin Housheng & Luo Peiyu *300 Questions on Qigong
Exercises* Guandong Science and Technology Press,
China, 1994

Hall, Judy with Dr Robert Jacobs *The Wise Woman –
a natural approach to the menopause* Element Books,
Dorset, 1992

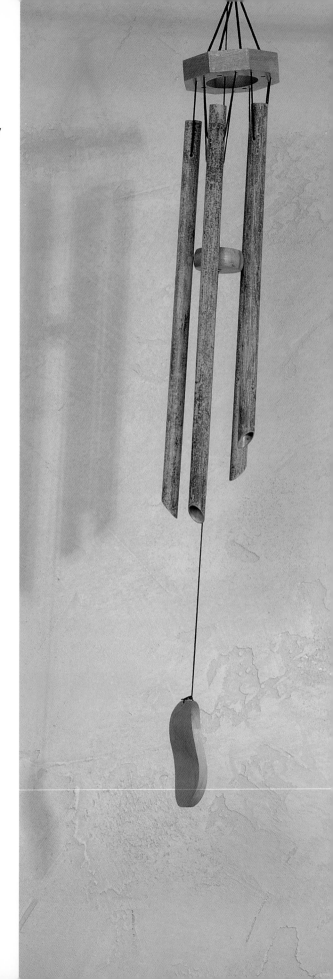

glossary

Baihui – 'The hundred meetings', acupuncture point on the Governor Channel, situated at the crown of the head

Conception channel – The main yin meridian running up the front of the body, from the *Huiyin* point to the bottom lip

Dantian – There are three *Dantian*, or centres of energy in the body. The lower *Dantian* is of primary importance to the Chi kung practitioner since it is where energy is stored for health and longevity

Dao-yin – An ancient term for Chi kung, which means leading the *chi*

Governor channel – The main yang meridian. It starts at the tip of the coccyx, follows the spine up to the crown of the head, and descends over the face, ending on the upper lip

Huiyin – Energy point located in the perineum, which is the meeting point of the Governor and Conception channels. In the Chi Kung posture, the *Baihui* and the *Huiyin* points should be aligned

Jing – Sexual energy – a yin form of *chi*

Laogong – 'Palace of work' located in the centre of the palm. This point is used to sense and transmit *chi*

Mingmen – The fourth point on the Governor channel opposite the navel

Shen – Spiritual energy – a yang form of *chi*.

Taiji – The philosophical concept of the unity of yin and yang

Taijiquan – More usually known as *Tai chi chuan*

Three treasures – The three essential energies of life: sexual (*jing*), *chi* and spiritual (*shen*)

Triple heater – A body function that does not have a specific physical correspondence. The triple heater controls water and energy in three areas of the body – upper heater (head and chest), middle heater (solar plexus to navel) and lower heater (lower abdomen)

the energy gates

Western	Chinese
Crown	*Baihui* – Heaven's Gate
Brow	*Yin Tang* – Decorating Place
Tongue	*Yinjiao* – Gum Crossing
Heart (front & back)	*Shan Zhong* (front) – Heart Palace, *Ling Tai* (back) – Spiritual Place
Navel/solar plexus	*Qi Hai* – Sea of Energy
Kidney point	*Mingmen* – Gate of Life
Perineum	*Huiyin* – Convergence of Yin
Centre of palms	*Laogong* – Labouring Palace
Centre sole of foot	*Yongquan* – Bubbling Spring (kidney points)

index